Animal Health

Animal Health

Health, Disease and Welfare of Farm Livestock

Second Edition

David Sainsbury

MA, PhD, BSc, MRCVS, FRSH, CBiol, FIBiol
Honorary Director
Cambridge Centre for Animal Health and Welfare
1 Leys Road, Cambridge CB4 2AP

**Blackwell
Science**

© 1983, 1998 David Sainsbury

Blackwell Science Ltd
Editorial Offices:
Osney Mead, Oxford OX2 0EL
25 John Street, London WC1N 2BL
23 Ainslie Place, Edinburgh EH3 6AJ
350 Main Street, Malden
   MA 02148 5018, USA
54 University Street, Carlton
   Victoria 3053, Australia
10, rue Casimir Delavigne
   75006 Paris, France

Other Editorial Offices:

Blackwell Wissenschafts-Verlag GmbH
Kurfürstendamm 57
10707 Berlin, Germany

Blackwell Science KK
MG Kodenmacho Building
7–10 Kodenmacho Nihombashi
Chuo-ku, Tokyo 104, Japan

First edition published 1983 by Collins
Professional and Technical Books
Reprinted 1986
Second edition published 1998 by
Blackwell Science

Set in 10/13 pt Bembo
by DP Photosetting, Aylesbury, Bucks
Printed and bound in Great Britain by
the University Press, Cambridge

DISTRIBUTORS

Marston Book Services Ltd
PO Box 269
Abingdon
Oxon OX14 4YN
(*Orders:*   Tel: 01235 465500
             Fax: 01235 465555)

USA
   Blackwell Science, Inc.
   Commerce Place
   350 Main Street
   Malden, MA 02148 5018
   (*Orders:*   Tel: 800 759 6102
                781 388 8250
                Fax: 781 388 8255)

Canada
   Login Brothers Book Company
   324 Saulteaux Crescent
   Winnipeg, Manitoba R3J 3T2
   (*Orders:*   Tel: 204 224-4068)

Australia
   Blackwell Science Pty Ltd
   54 University Street
   Carlton, Victoria 3053
   (*Orders:*   Tel: 03 9347 0300
                Fax: 03 9347 5001)

A catalogue record for this title is
available from the British Library

ISBN 0-632-03888-8

Library of Congress
Cataloging-in-Publication Data
Sainsbury, David.
    Animal health: health, disease, and welfare of
    farm livestock/David Sainsbury. – 2nd ed.
       p.   cm.
    Includes index.
    ISBN 0-632-03888-8 (pb)
    1. Veterinary hygiene.   2. Animal health.
    3. Veterinary medicine.   I. Title.
SF757.S24   1998
636.089–dc21   97-34605
                                          CIP

Contents

Preface to the Second Edition

The first edition of *Animal Health* was written in 1983. Much has happened since then to require the production of a new edition. Some totally new and important diseases have emerged, such as Bovine Spongiform Encephalopathy (BSE or Mad Cow Disease) in cattle, Avian Rhino-Tracheitis in poultry and an assortment of new respiratory entities in pigs. These are important yet in spite of a huge amount of research all of the examples I have given have defied a full understanding of their cause and control. The emergence of these diseases has in no way undermined the basis of this book which is one of prevention of disease or, more positively, the promotion of good health.

Another development in the past 10 years has been the much greater interest and concern shown by the general public in the methods of keeping animals and the maintenance of their good health and well-being. The interest by the public is to be applauded if it is based on a genuine knowledge of the methods actually being used. Regrettably, it must be said that this is generally not the case. The media does all in its power to scare the public with a combination of biased and inaccurate information, including allegations of cruelty to animals by farmers, misuse of medicines, dangers from residues in animal products, and risks of contracting diseases by eating aninal products. I hope fervently that this book will put the record straight and enable the reader to take a balanced and fair view of the situation whether the reader is himself involved in the livestock industry or is just a member of the general public who wishes to be informed. I have no personal axe to grind except the ever-present desire to see animals productive, healthy and kept under conditions of indisputedly good welfare.

D.W.B. Sainsbury

Preface to the First Edition

The aim of this book is to give a concise account of the factors affecting the health of livestock under modern conditions of husbandry and describe the most important diseases. Many of the classic livestock diseases have either been completely eliminated or kept under control with vaccines or drugs. What is happening now under the conditions of modern husbandry is that animals are affected by less obvious but nevertheless serious and often chronic infections which can have immensely damaging effects on productivity. In addition, farm animals are increasingly afflicted with metabolic disorders. These are the conditions which cause severely adverse effects on production and health due to partial or total collapse of the animals' metabolic processes when 'pushed' beyond their normal capabilities. And in the field of contagious diseases the new problem of 'viral strike' is emerging; many apparently new virus diseases, borne by wind or vectors, travel through areas, causing some quite devastating effects for a time, especially in the larger livestock units. In no few cases these diseases so cripple the enterprise that it never recovers.

In particular I hope I can convey to the reader the need for an understanding of the way the various diseases exert their effect and the overriding necessity for their absolute prevention to give to the farmer the incalculable economic benefits of healthy livestock. Good health is the birthright of all animals and such an ideal lies completely within our grasp.

D.W.B. Sainsbury

Acknowledgements

My sincerest thanks go to Grampian Pharmaceuticals Ltd, the C-Vet Livestock Division of this Company and Microbiologicals Ltd for supplying illustrations and general assistance. I am also grateful to the following for the supply of illustrations.

Messrs C.E. Davidson for Figs 1.10 and 1.11; Maywick for Fig. 1.15; Microbiologicals for Figs 3.3 and 3.4; Loddon Livestock Equipment for Figs 5.7, 5.8 and 5.9; Grampian Pharmaceuticals for Figs 7.1 and 7.2; Turbair Limited for 8.5 and 8.6; and Big Dutchman for 8.1 and 8.2.

In thanking Professor W. Holmes, editor of *Grass* and his publishers, Blackwell Science for permission to use Fig. 1.19, I would like to recommend that the reader studies this excellent treatise for a thorough grounding in such a vital agricultural topic.

Figures 4.1 and 4.2 and Tables 4.1 and 4.2 are Crown Copyright and are reproduced with the permission of the Controller of Her Majesty's Stationery Office.

I was helped throughout in the preparation of this edition by Joy Tuck, to whom I wish to express sincerest thanks, and from the publishers I received the invaluable and tireless assistance of Antonia Seymour and Robert Dyer and, as with all my books, the ever present guidance of Richard Miles. It is not so much a duty as a real pleasure to acknowledge their part in the production of this book.

Chapter 1

Health and the Environment

The changing health picture

Recent fundamental changes in farming practices have had a marked effect on the environmental influences on livestock health. These influences are now often the major factors affecting the economic viability of a farm.

In the first place, considerable advances in the control of animal infections have led to the effective elimination of many of the *traditional* causes of acute disease. This has been achieved by a combination of appropriate vaccine usage, good veterinary medicines, continually improving hygiene measures and the development of disease-free strains of livestock. These advances have made it possible to keep animals in much larger groups and more densely housed than hitherto but the results have by no means led to a gradual disappearance of infectious diseases altogether.

On the contrary, a number of complex diseases have emerged, which are difficult to diagnose and which are induced by a multiplicity of pathogenic agents. Whilst these agents may cause an apparent or 'clinical' disease, it is more likely that the effect will be less obvious and may only reduce the overall productivity of the livestock by, for example, slowing growth and reducing the food conversion efficiency. Animals may not die or even show any symptoms at all, so that the farmer may be unaware of what is happening unless he keeps very careful records and uses more than the usual degree of skill. It is also a very common phenomenon that intensive production on a livestock unit may start efficiently and effectively, but deteriorate so gradually with time that it is not noticed until the consequences have become very serious and control then becomes extremely difficult. The nature of these infections is of especial interest and concern because the environmental and housing conditions have a profound effect on their severity.

A second major problem is that of the *metabolic diseases*. These are a group of diseases that are caused intrinsically by the animals being called to produce an end product faster than the body can process its intake of feed. Enormous efforts are made to provide the right nutrients in an easily assimilated form but, as the metabolic disease is rather different from a deficiency disease, this does not necessarily work. In a way, the metabolic diseases are the inevitable outcome of the success in conquering the acute virulent diseases together with the advances made in improved genetics, nutrition and growth and productivity. Unfortunately, the capability of animals to keep pace with these advances has outstripped the normal functioning process (or metabolism) of the body.

A good example of this is provided by studying the growth of broiler chickens. When the industry started in earnest it took about 13 weeks to produce a bird weighing 2 kg, at a food conversion efficiency of approximately 3:1 (that is, 3 kg of feed to produce 1 kg of live weight). The hazards in growing these birds at that time were numerous but were largely related to contagious and infectious diseases – viral, bacterial, mycoplasmal and parasitic. Mortalities were high, often up to 30%, and of course the diseases played their part in slowing growth and damaging the food conversion efficiency. Now the position is quite different, it takes well under half the time for the birds to reach 2 kg: that is, about 5.5 weeks. Mortalities can average 4%, food conversion efficiency is 1.8:1 and contagious and infectious diseases are controlled largely by vaccines, medicines and good hygiene. However, we now have a plethora of the so-called metabolic or production diseases. For example, birds are affected with excess fatty deposition, causing degeneration of the liver and kidney and heart attacks. The skeletal growth cannot keep pace with the rate of muscle development so that many locomotor disorders occur, such as twisted, rubbery and broken bones and slipped tendons.

The types of disease

An important factor influencing the incidence of disease in livestock is the increasing immaturity of livestock. Improved performance has resulted in animals reaching market weight much earlier, whilst for genetic reasons, breeding animals are also younger on average than previously. Thus, in a livestock unit nowadays, there is usually a much higher proportion of young animals that are in a state of susceptibility to infectious agents whilst they are still developing the ability to naturally resist disease (natural immunity to disease) which normally takes place over a prolonged period (see Chapter 3). This difficult state of affairs is further exacerbated by the considerable size of many livestock units, in which the young animals may have originated from various parents of very different backgrounds. In many cases the young or growing stock have come in from widely separated areas, they may have no resistance to local infections and will therefore be susceptible to them, whilst at the same time contributing a new burden of pathogenic organisms to the unit they have entered. Altogether the modern livestock unit may present at any one time a confusing immunological state and the basic design and its management will influence the success or otherwise of disease control (Table 1.1).

Table 1.1   The disease pattern on the farm.
Bad husbandry + Primary disease agent + Secondary disease agents
$\qquad\qquad\qquad$ (often a virus) $\qquad$ (often bacteria or parasites)
= Subclinical or overt disease

Examples of bad husbandry
Overcrowding too many animals on a site
Mixed ages within a house or site
Excessive movement of animals
Poor ventilation and environmental control
Bad drainage and muck disposal
Insufficient bedding
Lack of thermal insulation in construction
Unhygienic or insufficient food and watering equipment
Absence of routine disinfection procedures
Faulty nutrition

It is appropriate to record the major groups of infections that contribute to these problems. Possibly the most widespread are the respiratory diseases. Many respiratory diseases are subclinical, have a widespread debilitating effect and are caused by a large number of different infective agents even in any one disease incident. They may not respond satisfactorily to vaccines, antisera, antibiotics or any other medicines, so that the only way to approach their control is by environmental and hygienic measures (Fig. 1.1).

Another significant group of diseases is enteric infections. These, as in the case of respiratory diseases, have many different primary causative agents, ranging from parasites to viruses and bacteria. The reasons for their increasingly harmful effects in recent years are not only those already listed earlier but also the general trend, for certain livestock, of eliminating the use of bedding, such as straw, which can be expensive to handle and store. Though the harmful effects of this may often be corrected by the use of good pen design, especially by the use of slatted or slotted floors, it is nevertheless rather more difficult to separate animals from their urine and faeces when the flooring is without litter, as the latter has a diluting and absorbent effect on the excreta and is also of great benefit to the comfort and welfare of the animals, which can contribute towards their health.

One may also consider the several important bacterial infections that have tended to increase in large intensive units. Examples of these are *Salmonella* and *Clostridia* bacterial spores, together with *Escherichia coli* and *Pasteurella*.

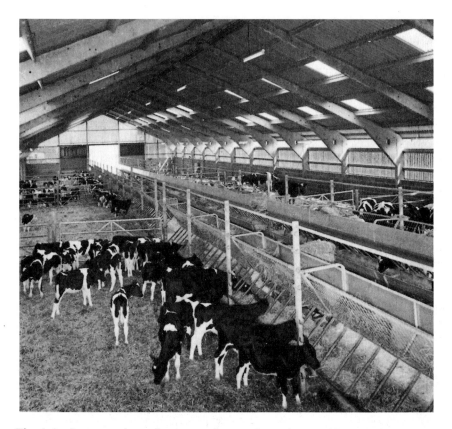

Fig. 1.1   Large numbers of young cattle reared together must be kept under ideal environmental conditions if respiratory disease is to be kept to a minimum. This building has a very large area of spaced boarding at the gables and sides to give good air flow.

Many forms of these organisms are normal inhabitants of the animal's intestines in small numbers but excessive 'challenges' causing disease may build up under unhygienic intensive conditions, encouraged by buildings with poorly constructed surfaces which cannot be cleaned. Recently in the UK and abroad there have been tragic outbreaks of a virulent form of *Escherichia coli* in man which may be traced back to the lack of cleanliness and hygiene in the cattle due to the absence of clean bedded areas.

Livestock unit size

In addition to the risks of the gradual build-up of disease-causing agents within a livestock unit, the dangers of livestock groups becoming too large must be borne in mind. In all parts of the world where the development of large units has taken place there has emerged a number of diseases chiefly of viral origin, which tend to 'sweep' like a forest fire through areas with a large livestock population, leaving a trail of devastation. Often there is likely to be considerable loss over a concentrated period, usually when the animal population either develops a natural immunity or when artificial immunities are promoted by the use of vaccines. It is now known that contagious and infectious particles can travel great distances from infected sites – certainly, distances of 50 miles have virtually been proven – but they may well travel much further than this. If livestock enterprises continue to grow in size then the dangers in this respect can only become greater. At the present time it is impossible to present soundly based objective advice as to the optimal unit size and in any event the factors that would lead to forming guidelines are highly complex. However, there is clear evidence that animals thrive less efficiently in large numbers, even in the absence of clinical disease (Fig. 1.2).

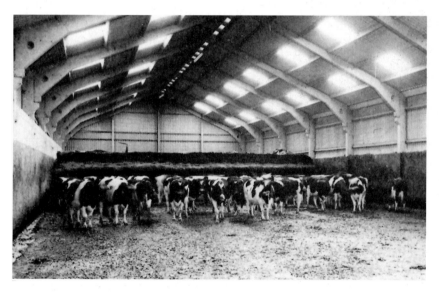

Fig. 1.2 A large cattle unit self-feeding silage. Such systems give many opportunities for cross-infection of disease and also bullying, so yield per cow is usually adversely affected.

Nonetheless, it should be made clear that it may be possible and economic to keep very much greater numbers of adult animals or birds together than young stock, since there is nothing like the same number of contagious disease problems after the difficult growing stage and its immunological uncertainties have passed.

As to the maximum number of livestock that might be kept on a site, it will be appreciated that this will depend on a number of factors, apart from health considerations. Figures have been proposed which attempt to allow for all factors and those suggested are as follows:

- ❑ Dairy cows: 200; beef cattle: up to 1000
- ❑ Breeding pigs: 500; fattening pigs: 3000
- ❑ Sheep: 1500
- ❑ Breeding poultry: 5000
- ❑ Commercial egg layers: 60 000; broiler chickens: 200 000.

Such figures can be no more than suggestions made in the light of experience on the farm. In due time more scientific evidence may be available to establish a better degree of accuracy. It is certainly likely that the figures will require constant adjustment in the light of new developments in husbandry, housing and disease control and especially with the anticipated trend towards the production of livestock free of specific disease, so-called minimal-disease stock.

Design essentials to minimise the disease challenge

In addition to the size of the livestock unit, a number of other basic items need to be considered in order to provide the bases of good health.

Depopulation

One of the most important concepts in disease control is ensuring the periodic depopulation of a building or a site. The benefits of eliminating the animal hosts to disease-causing agents are well understood and the virtue of being able to clean, disinfect and fumigate a building is also accepted. Nevertheless, in practice the whole concept of the 'all-in', 'all-out' policy is more complex than the preceding sentences would indicate. Periodic depopulation is extremely important for young animals but is less so for groups of older animals which have probably achieved an immunity to many contagious diseases. Much also depends on whether the herd or flock is a 'closed' one, with few or no incoming animals, or an 'open' one with a constant renewal of the animal population. If the latter is the case, then constant depopulation is of greater importance as there is little or no opportunity for natural immunities to develop and the regular removal of the 'build-up' of infection is of great assistance in ensuring the good health of the livestock.

The health status

The policy will also depend on the health status of the stock. At one extreme there are the so-called 'minimal disease' or 'specific pathogen-free' herds which have been developed to be free of most of the common disease-causing agents of that species. Here, depopulation is not so critical as the isolation of the animals from outside infections. Since this danger is very serious in most localities it is important to subdivide the animals in a unit into smaller groups, lessening the likelihood of a breakdown and/or enabling isolation and elimination of a group which may become infected. At the other extreme there are those units which have a constant intake of new animals from outside and of unknown disease status. In this case there is a constantly running risk – more usually, a near certainty – that some will be either clinically infected with, or will be carriers of, disease. Design specifications for such units should be quite different from those of the closed herd or flock so that defined areas of the unit should at least have groups of animals put through them in batches after which the area can be cleared, cleaned and sterilised. It is obviously preferable if the whole unit can be so treated since it ensures an absolute 'break' in the possible disease 'build-up' cycle.

Between these two extremes is the more usual case in which a herd or flock is of reasonable health status, although certainly not free of all the common diseases, and in which new livestock are added only occasionally. In such cases the precautions in the housing against disease 'build-up' and spread of infection can be relaxed, but there should still be proper provision for the isolation of incoming and sick animals.

Group size

An important means of putting the housing on the right lines is to keep the animals in groups of minimal size. This may seem to be an outdated policy that may eliminate all those advantages from automation that large units can give us, but this certainly need not be the case. If groups are small, it is usually easier to match the animals in them for size, weight and age, and it is well-established that growth under these circumstances is likely to be more uniform and profitable. Behavioural abnormalities, such as fighting and bullying, are also kept to a minimum – indeed they may be prevented altogether (Fig. 1.3).

Fighting amongst animals seems to be a highly contagious condition and under the most intensive management an almost casual accident that may draw some blood can escalate into a bloodbath. Pens which keep the animals in small groups will undoubtedly reduce the occurrence of such disasters,

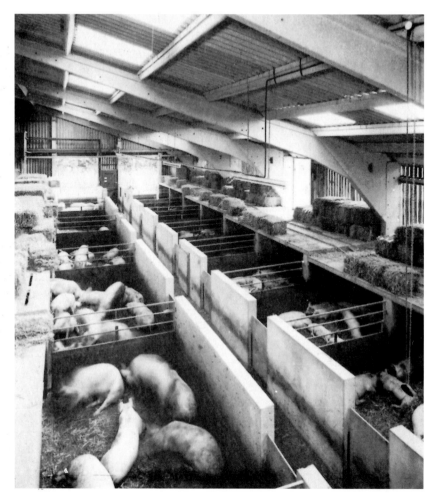

Fig. 1.3   Kennels within a large, generously ventilated building, a satisfactory combination of two housing systems, with the pigs in small groups.

and indeed with good management the removal of an animal that has accidentally injured itself or is off-colour and therefore prone to being bullied may stop the trouble before it has had a chance to get going.

There is yet another advantage in keeping animals in small groups. It is obviously good practice for a farmer to keep his livestock somewhere near the level that has been shown to be the densest that is practically possible for optimal productivity. For example, it is known that a broiler chicken will grow to its maximum potential at a stocking rate of about 15 birds per square metre. If birds are kept in a house to allow a density such as this, it means that they should spread across the house evenly, so that they fully occupy and use this area. In practice, however, this is rarely the case, especially when large numbers are housed together without any subdivisions at all. Hence, the birds, or such other livestock as may be at risk, crowd in certain parts of the buildings; this can lead to grossly overstocked floor areas. This is bad enough in itself but it has further unfortunate side-effects which may be seen as obviously in beef animals and dairy cows as in pigs and sheep. If livestock crowd excessively in certain parts of a house, this area is likely to become more polluted with dung and exhalations to an abnormal and harmful degree; the humidity becomes high, proper air movement is impeded and the animals may soon become ill. Sick animals feeling cold tend to huddle together more, so the vicious circle is perpetuated and there is seemingly no end to it unless some measures are taken to ensure a better distribution of the stock. When this problem arises under practical conditions it may often be impossible to subdivide the animals at once. An immediate move in the right direction of encouraging the animals to spread themselves more uniformly over the house can often be achieved by heating the building and intro-ducing some artificial heat. There are excellent portable gas radiant heaters and oil-fired and electrical blower heaters available which can meet heating requirements if no permanent system is installed. A temporary pen-within-a-pen may also help.

When animals are penned in large numbers, the effects of a fright caused by an unusual disturbance can be extremely serious. It is almost impossible to guard against all the extraneous sounds and sights that may affect the stock. The best safeguard, therefore, is to have the animals housed in small groups so that the effect of a panic movement will be more limited and will never build up into highly dangerous proportions. Guidance standards for stocking rates for housed livestock are given in Table 1.2.

Floors

The profound effect of the floor surface on the well-being of intensively managed livestock is well established. Previously, when bedding was almost invariably used and it was a cheap commodity to hand there were relatively few problems related to flooring. Now that the farmer, in an attempt to economically produce a comfortable and clean environment for his animals, must often turn to housing systems which have little or no bedding and often have slatted or some other form of perforated flooring, he finds himself facing a new set of problems. Although we are still far from being able to advise on the ideal floor, it is possible by choosing a good combination of surface, and bedding where used, to provide the animals with a comfortable, warm, hygienic and well-drained surface (Fig. 1.4).

The best solid flooring is usually based on concrete because when

Table 1.2   Guidance standards for stocking rates of livestock.

	Area per head (m^2)
Cattle:	
Cows – loose – housed	6
Calves to 3 months of age	2
Young cattle 3–6 months of age	3
Young cattle 6–12 months of age	4.5
Bull pen	30
Pigs:	
Sow – loose – housed	3.5
Sow – with litter	8
Boar	5
Weaner pig to 1 month old	0.18
Fattening pig 3–6 months of age	0.54
Sheep:	
Ewe	1.2
Ewe with lambs	1.5
Hoggs up to 30 kg	0.7
Lamb creeps to 5 weeks of age	0.3
Domestic fowl:	
Floor rearing – light breeds	0.12
Floor rearing – heavy breeds	0.18
Floor rearing – broiler breeders	0.24
Broilers to 6 weeks of age	0.06
Layers – deep litter	0.27
Layers – slatted floors	0.09
Layers – caged	0.06
Layers – strawyard	0.27

properly made and laid it is hard-wearing, hygienic and impervious to fluid. Where an animal lies directly on a floor without bedding, there should be an area of insulated concrete which is most often incorporated by using 100–200 mm of lightweight or aerated concrete under the top screed.

The surface of the concrete must not be so smooth that the animals slip or injure themselves, yet if it is too rough it can cause abrasions and injuries. A happy medium is not easy to find but is usually achieved by using a wood float finish and by tamping the floor lightly with a brush. Also, the slope of the floor is very rarely correct; there must be a nice balance between being steep enough to drain away liquids, yet not so sharp that the animals slip. With some animals the floor is made more comfortable by placing rubber or plastic mats on top; these are used with success with cattle, calves and pigs.

Some of the worst problems of injury, especially with cattle and pigs, have occurred with slatted or other forms of perforated floors. These have been particularly troublesome when the edges have been left too sharp or have

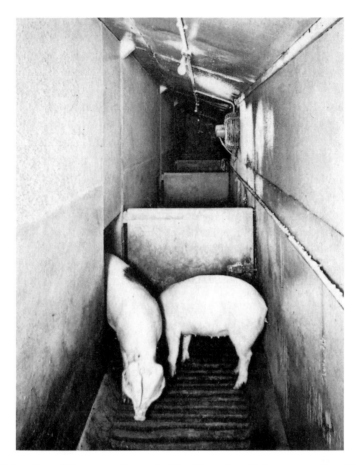

Fig. 1.4 Slatted floors can be a valuable aid to the efficient separation of animals from their excreta.

worn, leaving harmful protrusions. Great care is needed when choosing the correct flooring and making sure that it is maintained properly.

Building design sophistication

It is possible to be too naive and uncritical in our attitude to 'improvements' in the design of livestock buildings. If conditions in old and new buildings are compared, it can often be seen that the main advantages of new buildings are in economies of fuel and labour costs but not necessarily in productivity or health. New systems should certainly be carefully investigated under both practical and experimental conditions before they are advocated and adopted.

A housing classification in relation to health criteria

In a consideration of the relationship between health, environment and housing it is helpful to provide a classification that differentiates between the principal methods since they each require different schemes for environmental control. There are essentially three contrasting types of housing:

(1) *Climatic*, giving only a cover and protection from the elements, that is, wind, rain, snow and violent temperature changes
(2) *Controlled environment*, which regulates all parts of the micro-climate as completely as is required for the particular stock being housed
(3) *The kennel*, which is in a sense a half-way house between the other two and gives two environments in the one building, allowing some free choice for the animal in areas where they may go.

The methods of use of each of these types and their suitability for different countries, climatic regions and forms of livestock vary enormously and must be carefully defined. Some of the greatest errors in livestock housing are made by their incorrect application and it is vital to specify and understand these essential needs and differences.

Climatic housing

The climatic house is most suited to the adult which has developed a large measure of adaptability to climatic stress (Figs 1.5 and 1.6). The house can be

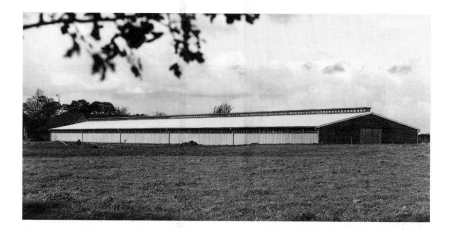

Fig. 1.5 A large 'climatic' building with an open ridge and generous side ventilation.

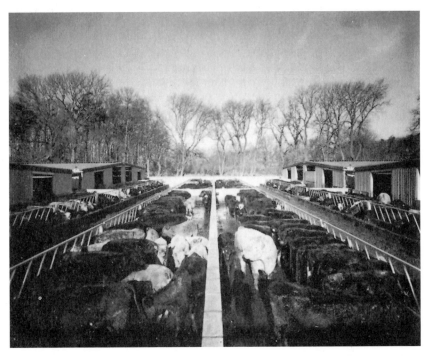

Fig. 1.6   A large cattle unit with outside feeding and inside accommodation in cubicles. Provided the site is well protected the free ventilation and open air feeding may assist in providing good health.

reasonably cheap, as it is basically only a cover, but because of the lack of control of the climatic, the space given to the animals must be more generous than in other forms of housing, especially since it is rare to have powered ventilation. In general, stocking densities tend to be half, or even less than half, of those for animals kept in a controlled-environment house. A major problem is created by agriculturists when they attempt to apply the highest stocking rates (suitable for the controlled-environment house) to the climatic house, as the building is unable to cope with the demands of the stock and poor productivity and serious disease problems can result. It is usually the correct choice of housing for cattle over 6 months of age, for sheep of all ages, for adult pigs which are bedded and very occasionally for poultry. Climatic housing often requires deep bedding, such as straw, for its success in cooler climates. This may be especially important because it is usual in climatic housing to have a surplus of air flow and to have little ventilation control. Even though this may be devised without causing draughts on the animals, it does involve quite fluctuating conditions so that the animals may need to have their own protection from the cold (Table 1.3 and Fig. 1.7).

Table 1.3   Essentials of good thermal insulation in an animal house.

1. High standard of insulation material, e.g. up to 150 mm thickness of glass fibre or 80 mm of polystyrene or polyurethene boarding. Even a 50% increase would not be out of place
2. Protection from damp penetration by good outer cladding and vapour-seal on the inside of the insulation, or a damp proof course in the floor below the insulation
3. Inner cladding must protect insulation and withstand disinfectants
4. Lightweight materials must not be compressed
5. Incorporation of air spaces on each side of the insulation increases the insulation value

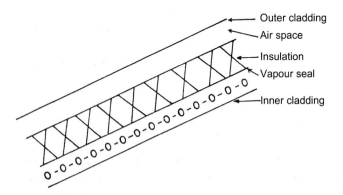

Outer cladding
Air space
Insulation
Vapour seal
Inner cladding

Fig. 1.7   Section through a well-insulated roof of an animal house.

The controlled-environment house

This type of building (Figs 1.8 and 1.9) is virtually the complete opposite of the climatic house. It may be used for all livestock but is especially appropriate for young animals, fattening pigs, chickens, animals of almost any age housed without bedding, and livestock which require an environment with light control. It is also most economically viable with animals which are largely fed concentrate food rather than substantial quantities of roughage, since the former is too expensive to be utilised as a form of energy. The housing is relatively expensive per unit area and sometimes extremely so in areas of climatic stress and where cooling devices are required. Because of this cost it is usually necessary to stock the buildings as densely as is practicable to make them economically viable; this can put the animals under a great health risk. To cope with the special requirements of this form of housing, the management needs to be highly trained and efficient: unless these criteria are satisfied, the controlled-environment house is frequently an unwise choice. The rewards, at their best, can be great but the dangers are also enormous and both the planning of the building and the management of the stock need to be of a higher standard than for the climatic house. A rather less intensive type of controlled-environment house is the Louisiana broiler house (Figs 1.10 and 1.11), a naturally ventilated and lit building

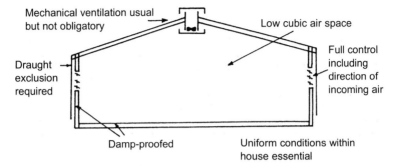

Mechanical ventilation usual
but not obligatory

Low cubic air space

Draught
exclusion
required

Full control
including
direction of
incoming air

Damp-proofed

Uniform conditions within
house essential

Fig. 1.8 A diagrammatic representation of the controlled-environment house.

which is now popular in many areas of the world but which was developed, as its name implies, in Louisiana.

Kennel accommodation

This is an increasingly popular system of housing (Fig. 1.12) which is a compromise between the climatic and the controlled-environment systems and attempts to combine the virtues of both at low cost. The essence of the system is that it keeps the animals grouped in separate pens, which promotes good health. The capital cost of the system may also be as low as any other.

The pens are sufficiently small to allow the animals to be closely confined, at least during their resting periods, without too great a danger from

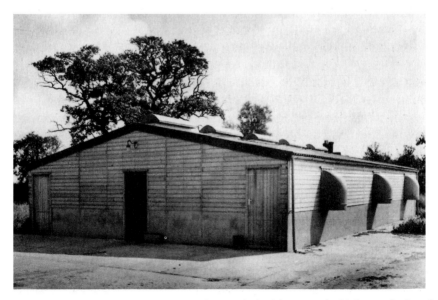

Fig. 1.9 Controlled-environment livestock buildings with high standards of thermal insulation, light control and mechanical ventilation.

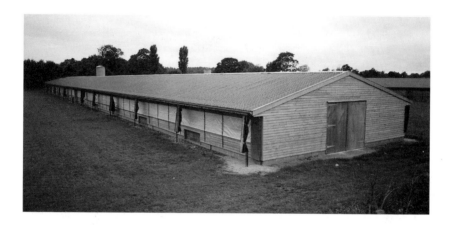

Fig. 1.10   Exterior of the so-called Louisiana naturally ventilated broiler chicken house. The ventilation is achieved by side curtains under the automatic regulation of a motor activated by a thermostat and a humidistat (courtesy C.E. Davidson).

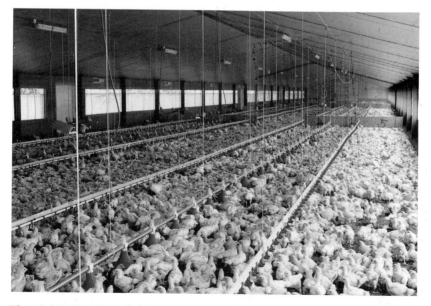

Fig. 1.11   Interior of the Louisiana broiler house showing the free interior allowing ventilation and movement of the birds (courtesey C.E. Davidson).

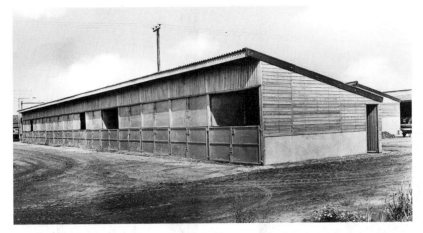

Fig. 1.12 The kennel or Monopitch house, with front ventilation only, controlled with ventilating flaps.

respiratory or other disease. This partitioned part of the accommodation approximates to the controlled-environment house. The close confinement makes it possible to keep the groups warm and draught free, generally by utilising their own body heat and by good insulation of the kennel and a limited cubic area (Figs 1.13 and 1.14). The separation of the pens from each

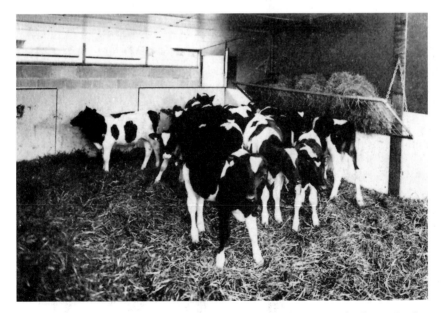

Fig. 1.13 A group of calves in a Monopitch house. There are only about 12 calves in this house which with plenty of bedding forms an ideal environment.

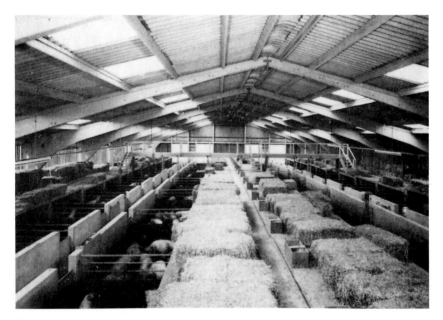

Fig. 1.14   Warmth in kennel housing is readily obtained by using bales of straw on the roof as a temporary measure. The straw can be used later for bedding.

other should be as complete as possible as this will limit the chance of a disease building up and spreading; where possible the partitions between sections should reach from the floor to the ceiling or roof.

The rest of the building comprises the 'yard' area which resembles the climatic house, the lack of environmental control in this area being acceptable because this is where the animals will be moving freely about and not normally lying down. The yard is likely to contain dung and so must be freely ventilated, usually by natural means. It is of benefit to the health of the animals if the muck is kept out of the warmer or closely confined resting area; this is easiest to achieve with the naturally clean pig but is also achievable, at least partly, with other livestock. Using good design to keep the muck from different pens from coming together until it has passed out of reach of the animals also improves hygiene and reduces the spread of enteric infections. In cold and exacting climates the outer section will be covered but in milder regions there may be no need for this and it can be left uncovered, which is beneficial to health, possibly to productivity and certainly to the cost of the operation.

The cheapness of this type of housing is due largely to the fact that the environment is controlled only where it is absolutely necessary. With controlled-environment housing becoming more and more expensive, there is no justification for the control to cover areas of effluent as this increases both the expenses and the risk of disease. The same reasoning can also be applied to service passages.

Table 1.4 summarises the use of the different types of housing systems.

Table 1.4 Ambient temperature ranges and housing systems suitable for housed livestock.

Type of animal	Ambient temperature range	Housing system
Adult milking cattle	Milk production optimum 10–15°C but little effect on yield from −7 to 21°C	Climatic housing usual and generally satisfactory
Beef cattle (from 3 months of age)	−7–15°C is the optimum range	Climatic housing appropriate but thermal insulation may be needed if bedding is absent
Calves	10–15°C at birth which may fall gradually thereafter. Higher temperatures (15–21°C) are normally used in veal housing	Kennel housing ideal, otherwise small units with some thermal insulation
Lambs	4–21°C	Controlled environments may be used if housing intensive, otherwise kennels or climatic housing satisfactory
Adult sheep	−7–30°C	Climatic or kennels
Adult pigs	4–30°C	Climatic housing suitable where bedding is used, but not with adults without bedding when minimum temperature should be about 15°C higher
Fattening pigs	15–27°C	Controlled environment or kennel housing required
Young piglets	21–27°C	Artificial heating needed to supplement controlled environment
Brooding poultry	30–35°C	Artificial heating, essential in controlled-environment housing
Broiler chickens	15–30°C	Artificial heating essential in controlled-environment housing
Laying poultry	15–24°C	Controlled-environment housing required with high standard of insulation or occasionally climatic housing with deep straw or other litter. Birds on free range need insulated housing

Artificial warmth as an aid to therapy

Under modern systems of management animals are often housed in very large groups. When an infection occurs, the illness usually produces a sense of chill in the body and there is a tendency for the stock to huddle together in an endeavour to keep warm. This is the animal's instinct but although it may achieve a warmer environment it will also aggravate the challenge of infection. The air around the animals may become vitiated with greater numbers of disease-producing organisms and the floor itself with higher concentrations of excreta, which may also have its quota of infection. One remedial measure that may be taken to correct this is to apply artificial heat, so discouraging a dispersal. In addition, if extra warmth is applied it will enable more ventilation to be used which will also tend to produce a healthier climate, and will be of especial benefit to livestock affected with respiratory ailments (Figs 1.15 and 1.16).

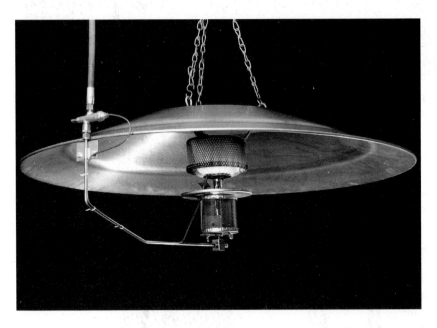

Fig. 1.15   Radiant gas heater ideal for the artificial heating of young or sick livestock.

It is not always possible, however, for the farmer to have an artificial heating source available; other paths may be taken towards the same end. Improved, possibly temporary, insulation will conserve the animal heat and raise the temperature. Temporary measures may be no more than making use of a few bales of straw around the animals. Another way of increasing

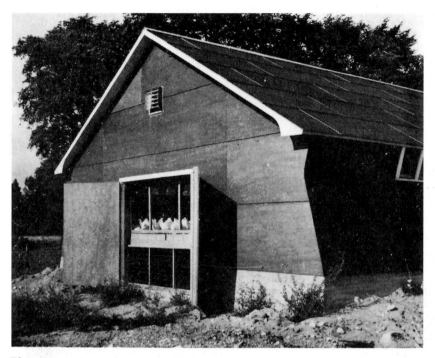

Fig. 1.16   Maintenance of a satisfactory environment may be enhanced by heat conservation, as in this two-storey prefabricated poultry house.

temperature does not mean necessarily the restriction of ventilation, which may do more harm than good, but involves more attention to the elimination of draughts and stale air pockets so that air flow is uniform throughout the building.

The importance of bedding

Within recent times there has been a trend for animals to be kept housed without bedding on slatted or perforated floors. These have one principal advantage in that they allow for the automatic disposal of dung and, if the design is good, they will keep the livestock clear of their own excreta. However, there may be serious disadvantages in eliminating the use of bedding.

Good bedding is an insulator of animals and is probably the cheapest way to retain heat (Fig. 1.17). The air temperature of buildings can more safely be lowered if bedding is used. When the bedding is straw it may be an acceptable, if not an essential, adjunct to the diet of the animal. The fibre may help digestion and create a sense of well-being. It keeps the animals

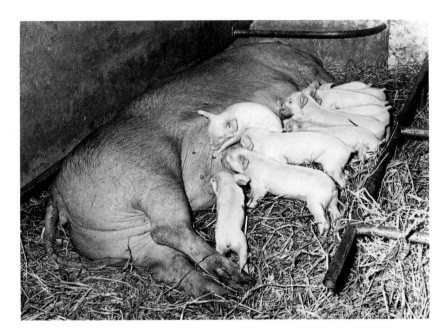

Fig. 1.17 The suckling pig. These 10-day-old pigs are in the cleanest of surroundings and have the comfort of copious bedding.

occupied and assists in the prevention of vices. Bedding also provides just about the safest flooring for the animal, so reducing the danger of injuries to the body and particularly the limbs. It is also much more difficult to keep the floor dry when no bedding is used, which can create a further chilling effect when the animal comes into contact with the wet surface.

It is also important to emphasise the health risk from undiluted muck which does not pass through slats but accumulates at some points, and the great risk to the respiratory system of man and animals from gases rising therefrom (see later in this chapter).

Not surprisingly, therefore, there has been a reaction against bare floors and slats, although it will be of little benefit if the amount of bedding used is inadequate or its quality questionable.

Isolation facilities

There is an urgent need for farmers to give better consideration to the isolation of sick animals; there are many reasons why this should be done. First and foremost isolation removes some of the dangers of contagion to the normal animals; it also makes it much more likely that the sick animal will recover without the unwelcome attentions of the other animals who will always tend to act as bullies. In nature the sick animal usually separates itself from the rest of the herd or flock but it is often impossible for the housed animal to do this. Also, under intensive management, more animals are likely to suffer from the aggression of their pen-mates and it is essential that such animals are removed to prevent them from suffering or being killed.

It is also easier, with an isolated animal, to give it such therapy as it needs and to give it any special environmental conditions, such as extra warmth or adjustments to comfort requirements. With these various items attended to there is a far greater chance of the patient recovering. It is an interesting but important observation, known to most farmers, that if you take 'poor doers', perhaps animals suffering from subclinical disease, out of a group, and pen them with more space and extra comfort, they may thrive without any further attention. Therefore, with the addition of suitable therapy, the cure may be completed.

Many modern livestock units completely ignore the provision of facilities to isolate animals and much greater attention should be given to this need. It is also an essential part of helping the attendant to do a satisfying job.

Health and the disposal of manure

The method used for manure disposal has potentially important effects on health, both human and animal. Whilst the smell of composted manure tends to be strong, it rarely travels far or creates a nuisance problem. There is little if any risk to the human or animal population from this form of manure under temperate climatic conditions as long as it is not placed too close to human dwelling places. Houseflies can breed in manure stacks and can produce undesirable concentrations in livestock or human housing.

Slurry, however, is quite a different matter. If placed straight on the land from the animal house or after holding in a tank anaerobically it has an extremely offensive smell. While masking agents are possible, they are too expensive at present to be considered economic. The worst smell comes from the pipeline and gun spreader, because the droplet size is small and light and particles may carry for considerable distances. Less smell arises from a tanker spreader because the slurry is much thicker and not spread by aerially dispersed small droplets. The most satisfactory way to prevent the slurry from causing offence is to treat it aerobically in some way before spreading. Human and animal health problems may arise from the spreading of slurry and particular dangers have been recognised from two groups of bacteria, *Salmonella* and *Escherichia*. In surveys it has been found that potentially pathogenic bacteria were able to survive up to nearly 3 months in slurry kept under anaerobic conditions. Whilst the particular bacteria studied were *Salmonella* species and *E. coli*, there is little doubt that more resistant organisms, such as *Bacillus anthracis*, *Mycobacterium tuberculosis*, *Clostridia* species and *Leptospira* species could survive as long or probably very much longer. It has been the author's experience that inhabitants of dwellings close to the dispersal of slurry may suffer from respiratory and gastroenteric problems whilst the slurry is being spread and in certain cases these may be persistent. Thus there are three possible hazards from the distribution of anaerobically stored slurry:

(1) Smells objectionable to the human population
(2) Hazards to human health
(3) Hazards to animal health.

If the slurry should enter a river or stream, the pollution may have far-reaching and infinitely more serious effects. It is thus essential for all enterprises with slurry as the disposal system that either the slurry is placed on land where it cannot be a nuisance or health risk or it is treated beforehand so that the risks are removed. Safe methods for disposing of solid dung and slurry are shown in Fig. 1.18. In the UK very heavy penalties are imposed on farmers who allow slurry to enter watercourses.

The dangers from gases in farm buildings

Hazards associated with gases in and around livestock farms have been evident, particularly in association with gas effusions from slurry channels under perforated floors. Numerous fatalities have been recorded of livestock, and even of man, due to gas intoxication. There is, in addition, mounting evidence that a concentration of gases in many livestock buildings may develop, affecting production adversely by reducing feed consumption, lowering growth rates and the animals' susceptibility to invasion by pathogenic microorganisms.

The most serious incidence of gas intoxication arises from areas of manure storage in slurry pits or channels under the stock, usually, but not always, associated with forms of perforated floors. The greatest risk arises when the manure is agitated for any reason, usually when it is removed. There is also an ever-present danger if a mechanical system fails and this is the only method of moving air in the house. Several cases of poisoning have been reported when sluice gates are opened at the end of slurry channels and the movement of the liquid manure has forced gas up at one end into the building. Sometimes the gases enter the building because bad management has allowed the slurry to accumulate too close to the slats.

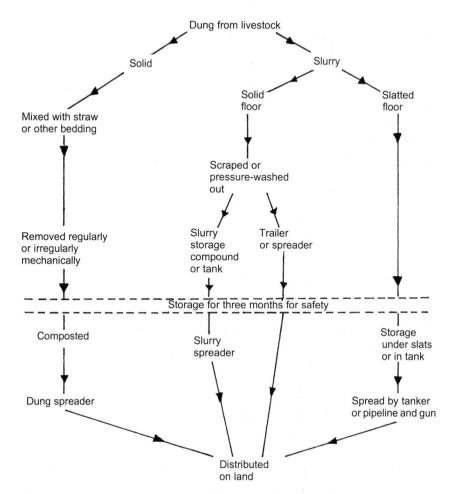

Fig. 1.18 Methods of disposing of dung safely.

High concentrations of gases, chiefly ammonia, may also arise from built-up litter in animal housing. This is most likely in poultry housing, since the deep litter system is the most commonly used arrangement with broiler chicken and poultry breeders. The danger has undoubtedly been exacerbated within the past few years, owing to the necessity of maintaining relatively high ambient temperatures in order to reduce food costs, while at the same time there has been good evidence that higher temperatures than before should be maintained for optimum productivity. Poultry farmers have often attempted to achieve such temperatures by restricting ventilation in the absence of good thermal insulation of the house surfaces and the result can be generally harmful, if not dangerous.

The most popular form of heating is by gas radiant heaters which are suspended from the ceiling. Well over half of all poultry housing is heated in this way and because the cost of gas appears to be improving in relation to that of other fuels, the system is being used more for pig housing and especially for piglets in the early weaning system. There is a risk that with inexpert use such heaters may be improperly serviced and the house so insufficiently ventilated that combustion is incomplete and toxic quantities of carbon monoxide may be produced.

The gases produced

The most important gases generated from stored manure are carbon dioxide, ammonia, hydrogen sulphide and methane; in addition there are traces of many organic compounds. Table 1.5 shows the limits of concentrations that are believed to be acceptable and these are expressed as threshold limit values (TLV) and given in parts per million (ppm).

Table 1.5   Acceptable limits (threshold limit value) for gases in the air of livestock buildings.

Gas	Threshold limit value (TLV) (parts per million)
Carbon dioxide	5000
Ammonia	50
Hydrogen sulphide	10
Carbon monoxide	50

Carbon dioxide

The TLV is about 5000 ppm. Concentrations of 2000 ppm can commonly be measured in normally ventilated controlled-environment houses. Fresh air contains about 300 ppm and more is released by respiration of animals and by manure decomposition. Most of the gas in bubbles coming from stored liquid manure is carbon dioxide. The gas in itself is not toxic but large quantities can contribute to oxygen deficiency and asphyxiation. Measurement of carbon dioxide is a good indicator of ventilation and is often used for this purpose.

Ammonia

This is an important gas in animal housing. Ammonia is released from fresh manure and during anaerobic decomposition of organic matter. The problem is less with slatted flooring than with solid flooring because of the high solubility of ammonia in water. A TLV for man of 50 ppm has been set to protect against irritation to the eyes and mucous membranes of the respiratory tract. Air containing 50–100 ppm can be inhaled for some hours without any apparent effect, at 100–200 ppm it induces sneezing, salivation and loss of appetite. It is known that in the chicken such levels slow growth rate, induce kerato-conjunctivitis and reduce appetite, but even in the worst ventilated of poultry houses it is unlikely that levels higher than 50 ppm would be found, although the modern practice of reducing ventilation to conserve heat makes the possibility distinctly greater.

Hydrogen sulphide

Hydrogen sulphide, with its highly characteristic smell of 'rotten eggs', is produced from the decomposition of organic wastes under anaerobic conditions. It is an extremely toxic gas and the TLV is 10 ppm. Dangerous concentrations can be released into a house if there is any form of agitation of stored slurry – concentrations of over 800 ppm have been found in livestock houses after slurry removal – and at this level unconsciousness and death in humans can result through respiratory paralysis.

Carbon monoxide

It is unlikely that carbon monoxide will appear in a livestock building other than due to the effect of incomplete combustion by gas burners. TLV is set at 50 ppm; there are a number of circumstances where this can occur. At certain times, as in brooding chickens or turkeys, the demands for heat are high but the need for ventilation is minimal. If management is careless, ventilators will be closed so that there is insufficient oxygen for the burners and substantial quantities of carbon monoxide, rather than carbon dioxide, will be produced. Also, the maintenance of the burners may be neglected so that deposits of debris build up around the air inlets to the burners and starve the oxygen supply.

As a general conclusion it can be stated that there is adequate evidence that gases cause intoxication in and around animal buildings but there is little information as yet on the precise magnitude of the problem. Reports in recent years have tended to highlight the more extreme and spectacular dangers when, for example, ventilation fails, slurry is agitated or the combustion by burners is incomplete. Very much less is known about the effects of sublethal concentrations of gases on livestock given a prolonged or even a lifetime's exposure to them. It has been the author's experience that in buildings with poorly designed perforated floor systems, which allow the introduction of gases into the living area, there may be serious morbidity from respiratory disease. In contrast to the known harmful effects of gases there is little evidence that dust has any deleterious consequences on health at the normal concentrations found in piggeries. Personal observation has concluded that a serious condition in poultry, ascites, is associated with poor ventilation or air circulation which has led to excessive ammonia accumulation.

Grazing management for health and productivity

The skilled management of grazing provides an adequate allowance of feed over the growing season, ensures efficient utilisation and maintains the productive capacity of the sward. There are several optimum systems of grazing management and they are briefly considered in this chapter in view of their health implications.

Grazing has a potential yield of dry matter ranging from 2000 to 25 000 kg per hectare and the quality in terms of metabolisable energy ranges from 6 to 13 megajoules per kg dry matter (MJ per kg DM). Thus there is an enormous variation in the nutritional value of different quality swards.

The implications for health of the type and management of the pasture are numerous. In other chapters the relationship is shown between hypomagnesaemia, bloat, parasitic gastro-enteritis, husk and liver fluke and the management of grassland. Emphasis needs to be placed on the dangers of overenthusiastic applications of nitrogenous and potash fertilisers and the resultant increased risk of hypomagnesaemia. Great care must also be taken when animals are moved on to pasture in the spring or off it in the autumn. Changes must be gradual since abrupt alterations can cause severe scour, metabolic problems and excessive effects from parasitic infestation. Overstocking of pasture and the running of young stock on pasture contaminated by the droppings of older animals also commonly create serious disease hazards. The practice of placing animals such as pigs and poultry on free range has not always been accompanied by sufficient understanding of the health risks if the land is overstocked or used for too long. In consequence there have been serious problems with parasitic and bacterial infection in particular.

The effect of the animal on pasture

The frequency and severity of grazing will influence the botanical composition of the pasture. Frequent close grazing encourages prostrate species and in British conditions results in a dense sward of perennial ryegrass and white clover. In contrast, infrequent grazing or cutting results in a less dense sward and encourages tall and stemmy plants, such as cocksfoot.

With rotational grazing management, the frequency of grazing is largely dictated by the length of the rotation cycle. On continuous stocking, frequency increases as herbage allowance declines.

Treading and poaching

Grazing animals exert pressure on the sward and compaction is more severe when the soil is wet. The effect of treading depends on the stocking rate, soil type and rainfall. Pasture species vary in resistance to treading, perennial ryegrass being one of the most resistant. In wet conditions, treading may break the surface sward, causing poaching, impairment of the drainage and seriously reduce the production of the sward.

Dung and urine

The daily production of faeces from stock varies, ranging from 2.5 to 3.5 kg DM for dairy cows; 1.2–2.0 kg DM for young cattle and 0.3–0.6 kg DM for sheep. Adult cattle faeces may cover 0.5–1.5 m^2 per day with proportionately smaller areas for smaller animals. A cow will void from 6 to 25 litres of urine daily.

Dung contributes considerably to the fertility of the soil but because of the uneven distribution and the low availability of the nitrogen (about 25% in the first year), the dung is of little immediate value as a fertiliser. Grass surrounding dung pats is often rejected. Urine, on the other hand, immediately contributes to plant growth and does not cause rejection.

Slurries from housed cattle, pigs or poultry are often applied. It is better if slurries are applied to arable land or grass to be cut for conservation. When applied to pasture they should be allowed at least 5 weeks before grazing and preferably longer. Great care should be taken in applying the correct quantities of slurry, expert advice should be sought depending on the type and condition of the land and the season of the year. Disease hazards have been referred to earlier in this chapter.

Stocking rate

Full production from pasture is achieved only when the needs of the animals and the productive capacity of the pasture are in balance. Stocking rate, which affects intake and animal performance, therefore has a major influence on pasture utilisation.

The stocking rate is normally expressed as numbers of animals per hectare for a given time period. A more precise measure is the weight, or for comparing animals of different sizes, the metabolic weight ($W^{0.75}$) per hectare.

The influence of herbage allowance in the short term and of stocking rate in the long term has been examined in many investigations. When herbage allowance is high animal production is at a maximum and as the allowance declines, the production per animal declines. Over the normal range, production per animal declines linearly with increasing stocking rate.

Efficiency of grazing

The herbage harvested by cutting either for one growth or for the whole season may be compared with that harvested by grazing.

Direct comparison with rotational methods of grazing is feasible since the quantities of herbage present before and after grazing can be estimated but comparison with continuous methods of stocking is more difficult. Efficiency of grazing varies from 50 to 90%.

Grazing systems

Grazing practices (Fig. 1.19) vary widely in the degree of control which they provide, their requirements for capital and labour and their influence on animal production and health and on pasture utilisation.

There has been a return by many farmers to simple grazing systems. The major distinction is between continuous and rotational methods. These methods have different effects on the swards. Continuous stocking tends to encourage the development of a dense sward with little bare ground and may encourage the maintenance of clover in the sward. In contrast, rotational methods, especially with long grazing cycles, tend to develop a more open sward which may be equally or more productive, but may be more sensitive to damage from poaching and less suitable for the maintenance of white clover.

Continuous stocking

This is when a group of stock has access to one area of pasture for the whole grazing season. It exists in its pure form only in extensive conditions where the stocking rate in relation to pasture production is low. There are, therefore, periods when grass growth exceeds the needs of the animals and the herbage becomes mature, dies and dilutes the available feed. Conventional hill grazing systems may approach continuous stocking. If the overall herbage allowance is high, grassland is underutilised, coarse grasses dominate,

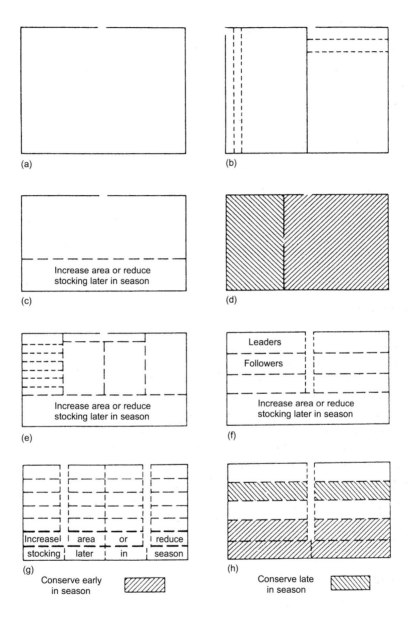

Fig. 1.19 Outline of grazing systems: (a) continuous stocking; (b) strip grazing (alternative methods); (c) intensive continuous stocking; (d) integrated grazing and conservation; (e) rigid rotational grazing; (f) leader and follower rotational grazing; (g) daily rotational paddocks; (h) flexible rotational paddocks. Permanent fence ———, temporary fence – – – –, movable electric fence - - - - -. (Reproduced by permission from *Grass*, edited by W. Holmes.)

shrubs or trees may establish and the nutritive value of the pasture deteriorates. If the overall herbage allowance is low, pasture is severely grazed, poaching or erosion may occur and the stock are undernourished and may be parasitised.

Intensive continuous stocking

The simplicity of continuous stocking which makes few demands on fencing, water supplies or labour, and allows the stock some choice in the selection of feed and shelter, coupled with the realisation that the stocking rate is the dominant factor affecting grazing output, has led to the widespread adoption of intensive continuous stocking, both with sheep and cattle. The stock are allowed access to an area of pasture for the early part of the season with numbers so adjusted that grass production and utilisation are in balance. To allow for the lower rate of production of grass towards the end of the year, stock requirements are reduced by the sale of fat stock and the removal to other pastures of dry cows or ewes, or of weaned calves or lambs. Alternatively, the area available may be expanded by including regrowth from areas previously cut for hay or silage, or by the inclusion of pasture sown in the spring which becomes productive in mid-season. These methods are widely used for all cattle and sheep. Risks of parasitic infestation are considerable if the pasture is overstocked.

Integrated grazing and conservation

This is also referred to as the '1:2:3' or 'full-graze' system. It combines some advantages of continuous stocking with some of rotational grazing. An area of pasture is allotted to a group of stock and divided in two in a ratio of between 33:67 and 40:60 by the grouping of existing fields or by dividing one large field. At the beginning of the grazing season the larger area may be grazed for 1 or 2 weeks. During the period of maximal herbage growth (mid-April to mid-June) the larger area is grazed while the smaller area, including any residues left when grazing ceased, is fertilised, allowed to grow for 5–7 weeks and then cut for silage. After mid-August the stock has access to the whole area. The area available is increased in the ratio 1:2:3, hence the name. It is simple to operate and economical on fences and water. It allows the stock freedom of choice and if surplus grass accumulates it can be cut and conserved. It also allows vigorous growth and build-up of root reserves and the fact that each area is free from stock for a period of 5–7 weeks helps to reduce the incidence of parasitic worms. The method is especially suitable for young growing cattle and can also be adopted for milking cows and suckler cows.

Rotational grazing

A greater degree of management control is provided by rotational methods of grazing which may also facilitate greater grass production, although the benefits are only in the order of 5–10%. The risk of parasitic infestation can be reduced to a minimum with rotational systems.

The *rotational or grazing cycle* is the total number of days elapsing from the beginning of one grazing period to the beginning of the next in a particular area.

The number of days within a cycle for which each paddock is unoccupied by animals is called the 'rest period'. Experience has shown that the grazing cycle in British conditions should be within 20–30 days.

Rotational grazing systems are classified as follows:

Rigid rotational grazing

Here stock spend a similar time in each paddock of similar size and move according to a predetermined timetable, irrespective of the defoliation of the sward.

A typical system is the Wye College system which includes four paddocks, each grazed for 1 week and rested for 3 weeks. For dairy cows it is preferable that each paddock is divided by a temporary electric fence to give a fresh allocation on each day of the week. The system is simple to operate and at appropriate stocking rates can achieve high performance with minimum effect. It is a system that promotes good health by reducing parasites.

Flexible rotational grazing

Adjustments to the variation in pasture growth rate are possible by varying the number of days within a paddock, depending on the quantity of grass present and/or conserving some of the paddocks. This system, however, is not usually so efficient as the rigid rotational system or 1:2:3 system because it is vital that in the first half of the season the cycle remains within 2–28 days. Attempts to achieve apparently efficient utilisation of the first paddocks to be grazed may result in the later paddocks reaching too advanced a stage of growth. It is also vital that the conservation of surplus paddocks is so arranged that a continuous supply of fresh grass for grazing is maintained.

Paddock grazing

This comprises either rigid or flexible rotational grazing with a large number of paddocks (20–30) where stock normally occupy each paddock for only 1 day.

Strip grazing

Moving an electric fence provides a fresh allocation of pasture daily. It is best organised within a cycle of rotational paddocks but may be employed in one field, for the early bite, autumn saved pastures and in times of pasture scarcity. In these circumstances a back fence should be provided so that the crop is not regrazed too soon. This helps pasture growth and reduces the risk of parasitism.

Leader and follower rotational grazing

Within the rotational pattern successive groups of stock of differing nutrient requirements may rotate. More than two groups complicate the operation and may restrict the recovery period. For ewes with lambs, two age groups of young beef cattle, or of growing heifers, the practice is useful. The animals which need the highest quality of diet should be the leaders. With sheep and lambs, forward creep grazing is the descriptive term. An eight paddock, 24-day cycle is preferred and lambs are encouraged to creep ahead, through specially constructed gaps in the fences, where they choose a high-quality diet and are possibly less exposed to worm larvae. Leader–follower systems always tend to reduce the incidence of worms because the younger animals are on clearer land for a longer period.

Chapter 2

The Animal Body

The skeleton

The skeleton is the part of the body which gives it its fundamental shape. It is rigid and permanent and consists largely of bone, but it also includes cartilage and teeth. With few exceptions, bones start as cartilage.

The skeleton also forms the structure to which the muscles are attached. The bones are composed largely of minerals: carbonates and phosphates of calcium and magnesium. The bone consists of a hard, outer part and a softer core – the marrow cavity – part of which is a honeycomb of spongy bone, particularly near the ends of the bones.

The backbone is the basal foundation of the skeleton and consists of small bones called vertebrae; articulation between these bones enables the animal to bend its back. The rest of the skeleton essentially articulates on the backbone and consists of the skull – made up of the cranium and the jaw bone – the long and short bones, separated by joints which form the framework of the fore and hind limbs, and paired ribs forming a hooped cage. Each of the ribs articulates with a vertebra at one end and fuses with the breast bone at the other end.

The typical long bones of the body consist of a shaft which is partly hollow and which is swollen out at the ends. The marrow cavity in the shaft is filled by blood vessels and soft fatty tissue. The dense bone consists of a matrix of white organic fibres impregnated and strengthened with mineral salts, chiefly salts of calcium and phosphorus. In this matrix are cells which are sustained by a capillary blood supply. Red blood corpuscles are formed in the marrow.

The skeleton functions to protect the organs of the body and to enable movement. The central nervous system is protected by the skull and vertebral column; the heart and lungs by the rib cage and the urinogenital system by the pelvis. In movement, it is the particular way in which muscles are attached to bones which enables the animal to move. Muscles always work in pairs because each muscle is capable of a pulling action. Thus one muscle pulls the bones in one direction and the opposite number in the pair pulls it back again (one is known as a 'flexor' and the other as the 'extensor').

The skeleton also serves as a storage for minerals, particularly calcium and phosphorus, which can be called upon when required, as in pregnancy, milk production and egg laying.

Joints (articulations)

Where bones adjoin and there is movement between them, the ends of the bones are coated with smooth cartilage to reduce friction and wear. The joint is lubricated by fluid secreted by the synovial membrane within the walls of the joint (Fig. 2.1).

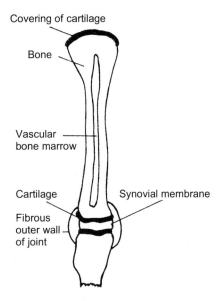

Covering of cartilage

Bone

Vascular bone marrow

Cartilage   Synovial membrane

Fibrous outer wall of joint

Fig. 2.1   A long bone and articulation (joint).

The bones are also held together by tough bands of fibrous tissue, the ligaments. The whole area of the joint is a peculiarly vulnerable part of the animal body and is often attacked by pathogenic organisms, or may be easily injured, especially in the very young or old animal. In the fast-growing animal the joints are also sometimes incapable of developing quickly enough to sustain proper movement of the limbs.

Correct growth and function of the joints is assisted by good nutrition, especially the provision of the correct quantities and balance of minerals and vitamins.

Teeth

There are three types of teeth: incisors, canines and molars. The incisors are the front teeth, then come the canines or tusks; the back teeth are the molars. All mammals have a set of temporary teeth which is succeeded later by the permanent teeth. Not all the molar positions are filled in the temporary set, the latter being known as premolars. As the numbers vary between different species, a dental formula is used which indicates the various teeth to be found on each side of the mouth for any species. In ruminants a hard pad, the dental pad, exists instead of the incisors on the upper jaw. The lower incisors tear herbage by gripping it between the lower incisors and the dental pad.

Judging the age of animals by their teeth is usually carried out by reference to the incisor teeth only. It is done on the basis of the time of eruption and subsequently the characteristics of the wear that takes place, which are well known for all farm animals.

The muscular system

The function of the muscles is to move parts of the body. Some muscles can be controlled at will and are called voluntary muscles, others operate outside the animal's control and are described as involuntary muscles.

The typical voluntary muscle has a tendon at each end with the body of the muscle in between. Tendons are composed of tough fibrous material because they have to take the strain when the muscle contracts by swelling laterally. The tendons of the muscles of the limbs are inserted into bone so, if one of two bones connected by a joint is stationary, the other must move when the muscle contracts. Many muscles are not attached to bone – for example, those which move the skin, and those which are involuntary in nature and move the stomach, intestinal walls and the heart.

The digestive system

There are clear distinctions between the digestive systems of single-stomached animals like pigs; ruminants, such as cows and sheep; and poultry, e.g. the domestic fowl.

In all cases, however, the basic arrangement is similar. The digestive system consists of a long tube, known as the alimentary canal, with a number of accessory organs associated with digestion, such as the liver and the pancreas. The canal starts at the mouth, continues as the pharynx or throat and then passes through to the oesophagus (gullet) which transports the food, which has in most cases been chewed or masticated, to the stomach or stomachs. The food then goes on to the small or large intestine for the major processes of digestion and, finally, undigested material is voided at the anus (or cloaca in the bird). In the process of dealing with food there are the processes of mastication – breaking up the feed – which is done by the teeth in mammals but in the gizzard in the case of chickens. The food is then digested by chemicals which break down the proteins, carbohydrates and fat in the food into products that are simple enough to be absorbed through the intestinal wall. Digestion is brought about by enzymes which are secreted by glands such as the pancreas and pass into the alimentary canal.

All the organs of the body are delicate and need protection, either as they move against each other or as material passes along the alimentary canal. Both protection and lubrication is supplied by membranes which line the organs.

The lining of passages which communicate with the exterior, such as those in the alimentary canal or respiratory system, is called mucous membrane. Linings which cover surfaces closed from the exterior are called serous membranes. Membranes vary considerably in their strength and thickness: for example, the mucous membrane lining the mouth is tough because the food may be quite coarse and damaging, whereas that lining the intestine is much thinner because the food is now soft and wet. All mucous membranes secrete mucus, a slimy lubricant, but in illness the absence of secretion may be an early feature. The serous membranes lining the body cavities are the peritoneum around the abdomen and its organs, the pleura around the lungs and the pericardium around the heart.

An outline of the digestive process

The single-stomach animal

Food passes into the mouth, is masticated with teeth, moved with the tongue and is exposed to secretions from the salivary glands containing the enzymes which commence the process of digestion. At the rear of the mouth is the pharynx, which has several openings (including that from the nose), and at the base is the entrance to the trachea (windpipe), which leads to the lungs, as well as the entrance to the gullet or oesophagus (Fig. 2.2). The food passes down the oesophagus to the stomach; here food is further digested and stored and is released into the intestines in controlled amounts.

The intestines are up to 30 metres long in the pig and are divided into the small intestine (duodenum, jejunum and ileum) and large intestine (caecum, colon and rectum). Most food is actually absorbed from the small intestine. Enzymes pass from the pancreas into the duodenum and from the liver via the bile gland and duct. In the large intestine much of the water is absorbed, leaving relatively dry faeces to pass out via the anus.

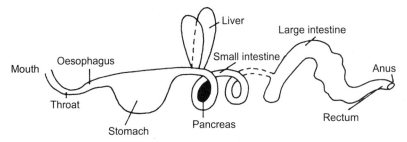

Fig. 2.2   Alimentary system of a pig.

The ruminant

The ruminant (Fig. 2.3) has four stomachs. The first is the large rumen, which can occupy up to half the abdomen and in cattle holds as much as 250 litres. From here the food passes to the *reticulum*, then the *omasum* and finally the *abomasum*, which is the organ which has the same function as the stomach of the single-stomach animals.

The complexity of this system enables the ruminant to deal with coarse and fibrous feed. Food is swallowed first without any real mastication but regurgitated later in mouthfuls and ground between the molar teeth.

· There is great activity all the time in the ruminant's stomach, producing much heat and gas, with constant eructations of the latter.

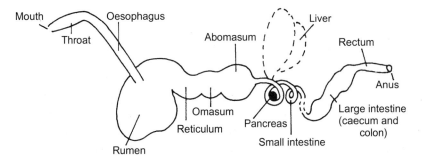

Fig. 2.3   Alimentary system of a ruminant.

The fowl

The fowl's digestive system is different (Fig. 2.4). The beak gathers the food material and at its edges are tactile cells by which the bird decides whether it will accept the food or reject it. The food is swallowed whole, with a little saliva added, passes down the oesophagus to the crop, which is only basically a container for bulky food. Here the food passes to the proventriculus,

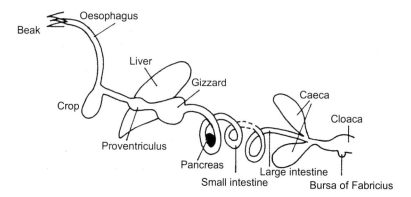

Fig. 2.4   Alimentary system of a fowl.

which secretes hydrochloric acid and pepsin, and then to the gizzard – a strong muscular organ which contracts powerfully, reducing the contents to a thick paste-like mass with the aid of the insoluble grit present within it. The food then passes to the small and large intestines and finally the faeces go to the cloaca, whose functions also include the excretion of urine, the acceptance or delivery of semen and the passage of the egg.

The respiratory system

The respiratory system's function is essentially to enable oxygen to be brought into the blood and remove the carbon dioxide and water from it (Fig. 2.5).

The fresh air that is so vital for life passes through the nostrils. Mammalian nostrils are lined with turbinate bones which are thin plates arranged in cylindrical fashion. These bones are lined with highly vascular mucous membranes and are also equipped with small hairs (cilia). The vascularity helps to warm air before it enters the lungs and the cilia help to trap dust and germs. However, their vulnerability makes the turbinate bones very susceptible to damage of the kind epitomised in atrophic rhinitis in pigs.

At the back of the throat is the larynx which is the gateway to the trachea. The trachea is constructed largely of rings of cartilage which safely maintain its rigidity. When the trachea reaches the lungs it divides into two bronchi which then divide and subdivide into numerous branches known as bronchioles which end in sacs known as alveoli, where the exchange of oxygen and carbon dioxide and water vapour takes place. The lungs also provide a suitable site for the settlement and multiplication of many pathogenic organisms.

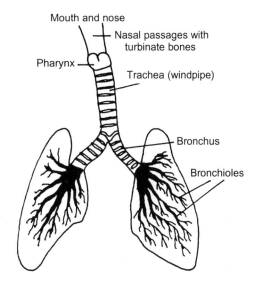

Fig. 2.5 The respiratory system.

The circulatory system

The blood is the transport medium for gathering oxygen from the lungs and the food products absorbed from the intestines, and also releasing carbon dioxide through the lungs and other waste products chiefly through the kidneys. Blood also regulates the heat of the body.

The blood circulates via the heart, arteries, veins and capillaries. Arteries convey the blood away from the heart; veins bring blood back towards the heart.

The main artery leaving the heart, the *aorta*, distributes the blood to all parts of the body via various branches (Fig. 2.6). Arteries go on dividing to form arterioles and, eventually, very small capillaries which form the links in the tissues between the arterioles and the venules, which are the first stage of the venous system whose function is to return blood to the heart. It is by means of the capillaries that the exchange of gases, nutrients and waste products takes place. From the venules, the blood passes to the veins which eventually take all the blood back to the heart.

Arteries are strong, elastic, muscular tubes as they must withstand the powerful force of the heart beat which drives the blood through them, while veins have a passive role of conveying the blood back to the heart. The arteries supplement the force of the heart and expand and contract to help the blood on its way.

Where the arteries leave the heart one-way valves prevent the blood flowing backwards as the heart expands for its next quota of blood. These are

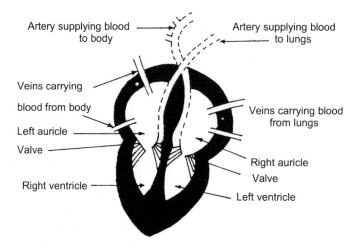

Fig. 2.6   The heart.

the only arterial valves but valves are frequent in veins to prevent the blood flowing back away from the heart. Arterial blood which is oxygenated is bright red, while venous blood is darker.

The heart and lungs

The powerful heart is situated nearly in the centre of the thorax (chest) and consists of four cavities – two on each side. There is no direct contact between the left and right sides, except in the fetus when the functionless lungs are short-circuited. The upper cavities are known as the auricles and the lower, separated by valves, as the ventricles.

Blood from the whole body enters the right auricle and passes through the one-way valve to the right ventricle as the auricle contracts and then, as the ventricle contracts, blood is forced into the pulmonary artery leading to the lungs. After passing through the lung capillaries, where carbon dioxide is released and oxygen collected, the blood travels via the pulmonary vein to the left auricle. Contraction of the two sides of the heart is simultaneous and from the left ventricle blood is pumped via the aorta to all parts of the body.

Blood

Mammalian blood is composed of fluid and cells. The fluid, blood plasma, is a solution of nutrients and salts and includes carbon dioxide, mostly in the form of bicarbonates.

The red colour is due to the red blood cells, present at the rate of about 6–10 million per cubic millilitre. They have no nucleus except in the youngest stages and their total life in the blood stream is about 6 weeks. The red colour is a protein called haemoglobin and this contains iron. Haemoglobin readily takes up oxygen (from the lungs) and gives it up to the tissues as required.

White blood cells are present in the blood at the rate of about 8000 to 17 000 cells per ml^3 (ruminants contain much less than pigs). There are many different types and their main function is to protect the animal against invasion by pathogenic microbes. The two main types of white blood cells are lymphocytes and the polymorphonuclear leucocytes: the latter can alter their shape and they will pass through the walls of capillaries in areas of inflammation and engulf invading organisms in order to digest them.

There are also blood platelets – about 200 000 per ml^3 – small cells which are concerned with the clotting mechanism. If bleeding occurs the platelets fracture and release an enzyme, resulting in the formation of fibrin, a stringy material which adheres to the walls of wounds and enmeshes escaping blood cells. The fibrin contracts and draws the cells together, thus tending to seal the wound and stop the haemorrhage.

The lymphatic system

Lymph is a cloudy fluid produced in the tissue spaces from the blood plasma which passes out of the capillaries to assist the function of the individual cells. The tubes of the system join up as the veins do but they are much smaller. Ultimately lymph finds its way into the anterior vena cava near the heart. Along the lymphatics are the nodes where lymphocytes are generated. Any foreign material not dealt with at the site of entry will find its way along the lymphatics and each lymph node acts as a barrier to further advance. Invading bacteria will usually have to overcome several of these barriers before reaching the bloodstream for general circulation. The lymph nodes become enlarged, tender and inflamed when dealing with an invasion.

The urinary system

The urinary system (Fig. 2.7) consists in the mammal of two kidneys, two ureters, the bladder and the urethra. The kidneys are situated under the lumbar vertebrae and are extremely well supplied with blood. Their function is to remove all the waste products of metabolism which are carried away in the urine. The exchange of products takes place by diffusion. This occurs in many glomeruli situated in the outer part of the kidney, the cortex. A glomerulus (Fig. 2.8) looks like the head of a flower in cross-section. Capillaries ramify in the glomerulus and the space around the capillaries is

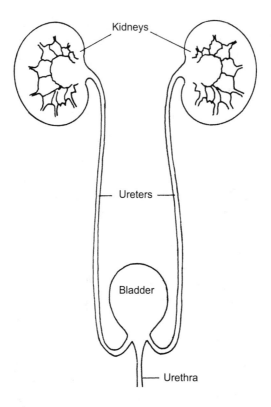

Fig. 2.7 The urinary system.

the beginning of a urinary tubule which leads to the centre of the kidney, from where a tube known as the ureter leads to the bladder. Water containing the waste products of metabolism and minerals in solution passes from the blood capillaries of the glomeruli into the urinary tubules.

Urine is continually produced in the kidneys and trickles down the ureter on each side to enter the bladder situated on the floor of the pelvis. The bladder is a storage organ composed of highly muscular tissue and is pear-

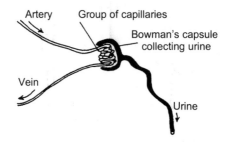

Fig. 2.8 Schematic diagram of a section through a glomerulus.

shaped, with the narrow end pointing hindwards and ending in a sphincter muscle which leads into the urethra. The sphincter muscle is normally closed but as the bladder becomes distended nerve impulses lead to the releasing of the sphincter and contraction of the muscle of the bladder to assist in the elimination of the urine.

The bladder leads to the urethra. The female urethra is short with a wide passage and opens into the vagina just above the bladder. The vagina is shared by the genital system which opens to the exterior through the vulva, an opening situated immediately below the anus.

The male urethra is a long, narrow tube directed backwards from the bladder along the floor of the pelvis and then curled down and forward under the pelvis to continue in the substance of the penis.

The genital organs

The male

Sperm for reproduction is produced in a pair of testicles which are situated in the scrotum (Fig. 2.9). Nerves and blood vessels serving the testicles enter the scrotum through the spermatic cord which also includes the vas deferens, the tubes along which sperm travel from the testes. In farm animals such as the bull, ram and boar, the scrotum is suspended under the abdomen, although in the boar the scrotum is held close to the body.

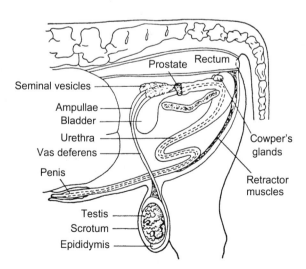

Fig. 2.9 Reproductive system of a male mammal.

The testicles orginate inside the abdomen of the foetus and travel down sometime near parturition through an opening between muscles on each side. In passing out of the abdomen into the scrotum, each testicle takes with it a fold of peritoneum. Thus there is a risk of hernia, i.e. the extrusion of abdominal contents (in this case intestine) into the scrotum. Hernia is most common in the pig. In some cases the testicle fails to enter the scrotum; it may come later or be permanently retained in the abdomen. A male animal with this defect is called a *rigg*. The production of fertile spermatozoa in most farm animals is adversely affected by high temperatures, especially as the testicles are located outside the abdominal cavity. Consequently the male of several species can become relatively infertile in hot weather.

The vas deferens, after leaving the testicles and passing up the spermatic cord, continues over the bladder to enter the urethra before it enters the penis, which is normally held within the prepuce – a fold of protective skin. The penis has much elasticity and contains spaces within it which are part of the blood circulatory system. Under sexual stimulus these spaces become engorged with blood, resulting in a substantial lengthening and stiffening of the penis so that it protrudes from the prepuce – an essential process in copulation.

The female

Ova, the primary female cells in reproduction, are produced in the paired ovaries situation high in the abdominal cavity. The ova are small bodies varying in size and shape during the sexual cycle. In the substance of the young ovary are many follicles, each containing one large cell, the ovum. Most of the follicles are at any time quiescent but enlargement occurs before any follicle bursts to release an ovum into the fallopian tube or oviduct, a much convoluted narrow tube which leads to the uterus (or womb).

The uterus is an organ of greatly variable size, for it is here the young develop before birth. The uterus has a cervix (the neck) and body and two horns. Each fallopian tube enters a horn. The two horns form the main part of the uterus and one or both become greatly distended during pregnancy. The horns join to form the short body and the cervix is the area of the complex sphincter muscle which is normally closed, opening slightly during oestrus and subject to great distension at the time of parturition. The wall of the uterus is muscular. During pregnancy the muscle increases in size and power. The fetal membranes are attached in various ways to the uterus and by this means receive nutrients.

Passing back from the cervix is the short but very distendable vagina which opens to the exterior at the vulva (Fig. 2.10).

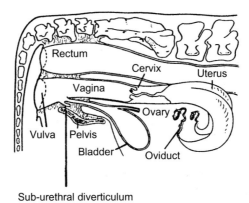

Fig. 2.10 Reproductive system of a female mammal.

Reproduction

At puberty animals become sexually active. The male seeks the opportunity for mating and the female commences the cyclic period of oestrus or heat when she is receptive to the male. As puberty approaches, the secondary sex characteristics develop. This is most noticeable in the features and shape and form of the head, but the whole male frame is bigger and somewhat coarser.

Oestrus is the state of heat when a female will accept a male. This happens in regular cycles. The cycle is about 21 days in the cow, 17 days in the ewe and 21 days in the sow. Oestrus itself lasts up to about 24 hours in the cow and up to 2 days in the ewe and sow. Oestrus is controlled from the ovaries, the animal coming into oestrus as a follicle approaches maturity just prior to releasing an ovum into the fallopian tube. After rupture of the follicle slight bleeding occurs and a clot forms in the ovary; this clot shortly forms the corpus luteum. The corpus luteum grows during the first part of the oestrus cycle and disappears before the next oestrus. If the animal becomes pregnant the corpus luteum continues to grow slowly and only recedes in the second half of the pregnancy. The presence of the corpus luteum inhibits oestrus and delays the development of any more ovarian follicles.

Cows and sows have oestrus cycles at all seasons but in sheep the oestrus cycles are limited to a definite season. There is considerable variation in the factors that induce a return to oestrus cycles after parturition.

The reproductive system of the fowl is essentially the same as in the mammal but with certain notable differences. The testes of the male remain within the abdominal cavity near the kidneys. In the hen, only one ovary, the left, develops and becomes functional. In the functional female the ovary

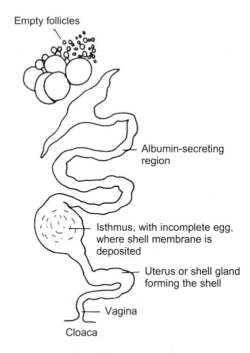

Empty follicles

Albumin-secreting region

Isthmus, with incomplete egg, where shell membrane is deposited

Uterus or shell gland forming the shell

Vagina

Cloaca

Fig. 2.11   Ovary and oviduct of a chicken (after Romanoff).

contains five or six large developing egg yolks (follicles) and a large number of small white follicles which represent immature, undeveloped yolks. The large convoluted oviduct (Fig. 2.11) is the site of egg white secretion, shell membrane and egg shell formation. As the yolk passes down the oviduct, the remainder of the egg is formed and then is 'laid', after which most of the development of the embryo takes place if the fertilised egg is 'incubated' for 21 days at about 37.5°C.

Sexual activity in birds is stimulated by increasing amounts of light, as in springtime, whereas decreasing amounts, as in the autumn, tend to put birds off laying and lead to a moult. Most hens will produce about 150 fertile eggs in a season.

Signs of oestrus vary. In the ewe they are slight unless a ram is present and he is probably attracted by smell. The sow when in season becomes quiet and it is possible for the boar to sit on her back, whereas at other times she is not likely to accept this. An important essential with pigs is to place boars within sight, sound and smell of the sows.

In cows there are certain signs of heat. One cow may ride another, but either may be on heat. The cow on heat is restless, may try to break out and is noisy. The vulva is usually swollen and there is a stringy mucous discharge.

Pregnancy

At mating the tadpole-like sperms move vigorously up the female tract into the fallopian tube where, if fertilisation is to take place, the sperm and ovum (the female egg) join together to form the embryo. During pregnancy certain changes take place. Oestrus cycles cease. Abdominal enlargement takes place. Various techniques exist to determine very early pregnancy, including palpation, hormone determination and sonic recorders.

The upper mammary glands also gradually enlarge in preparation for the supply of milk. Pregnant animals also tend to put on weight gradually and their temperament often improves and they become more docile.

The nervous system

The central nervous system is the name given to the brain and spinal cord. The rest of the nerves are described as being peripheral. The cells of the nervous system have processes which carry impulses or messages. There may be several short processes to receive messages but only one process takes impulses from the cells and this may be extremely long, extending right down a limb. These long processes are extremely fine individually, but large numbers of them are bound together to form the nerve which can be seen with the naked eye.

All conscious action and thought is centred in the right and left hemispheres of the brain. Subconscious control may be affected from the cerebellum at the back of the brain, below which the medulla oblongata leads into the spinal cord, which runs through the spinal column.

Nerves leave the brain to serve the head and the special organs of sight, hearing and smell. Branches leave the spinal cord behind the arch of each vertebra in pairs, one on each side (Fig. 2.12). The main nerve trunk of the limbs, such as the radial in the fore limb and the sciatic in the hind limb, are derived from several branches of the spinal cord. The nerves in their bundles are of two types: *afferent* nerves bringing messages into the brain, sensations of touch and temperature; and *efferent* nerves taking messages from the brain which result in action. All parts of the body are served by both types of nerves.

The autonomic nervous system

In addition to the nerves serving centres in the brain, a whole system of nerves governs the involuntary activities of the body (Fig. 2.12). These autonomic nerves are linked to each other and have connections with the

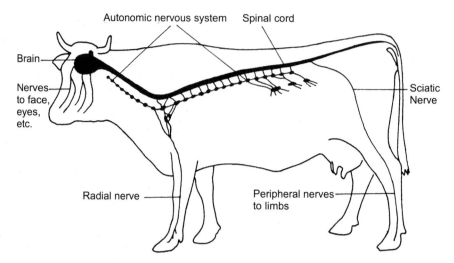

Fig. 2.12   Diagrammatic representation of the central nervous system and auto-nomic (sympathetic and parasympathetic) nervous system.

spinal cord. They control the activities of glands, the involuntary muscles of the digestive and other systems, the heart muscle and the pupil of the eye.

The autonomous nerves are in two groups working antagonistically to meet the varying needs of the body. One group, the sympathetic nervous system, produces effects similar to those produced by the hormone adrenalin: it reduces the activity of the digestive system, stimulates the heart muscle and tends to concentrate the blood in the areas of action. The sympathetic nerves are therefore in the ascendancy in an emergency. The other group, the parasympathetic nerves, stimulate muscular and glandular activities in the digestive system, urinary and sexual activity and have a depressing effect on the heart muscle. Afferent nerves from all over the body can bring impulses resulting from touch, pressure, temperature and pain, but certain organs are responsible for special senses which are of great importance to the animal – the eyes, the ears and the centres responsible for smell and taste.

The skin

The skin is the protective outer layer of the body. It is richly supplied with nerve endings responsible for sensations of touch, heat, cold and pain. The skin is continuous with the mucous membranes at all the natural orifices of the body. It varies greatly in thickness and toughness and sensitivity, depending on the needs of the situation. The outermost layer of the skin, the epidermis, is a thick mass of cells with neither blood supply nor nerve endings. These cells are continuously being shed. Underneath is the true skin, the dermis, with both blood and nerve supply. It contains hair follicles (Fig. 2.13) together with sebaceous glands which produce an oily protective material. Sweat glands which assist in the heat-control mechanism, are also present in the skin.

Hair and wool are modifications of skin; they are hard protein substances which serve as a means of protection. Hair is continually being shed and thicker hair will grow to respond to cooler conditions. Hoof and horn are also modifications of skin composed of hard protein.

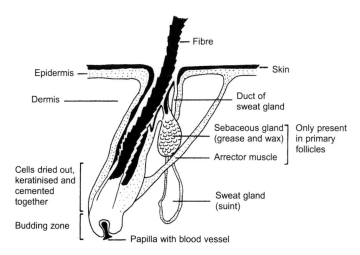

Fig. 2.13   Cross-section of a hair follicle, also showing structure of skin. (Courtesy of Dr D.C. Dalton.)

The endocrine organs

The endocrine organs (also called ductless glands) produce secretions but instead of being led by ducts to their point of use, they pass directly into the blood stream where they can travel to all areas as required. These secretions are called hormones. The glands and their main functions are described in the following sections.

Thyroid gland

The thyroid gland is situated in the neck close to the larynx. Thyroxin, the hormone it produces, contains iodine, which is an essential element in its production. Thyroxin is a general long-term metabolic stimulant, it is a master hormone in its effect on metabolism. A deficiency of thyroxin results in a fat, sluggish individual that loses its hair. Excessive thyroxin increases growth rate, activity and appetite.

Hypothyroidism occurs in areas of low iodine, such as Derbyshire. In these areas iodine supplements are necessary for the thyroid gland to function correctly.

Parathyroid glands

These are very small glands situated within the substance of the thyroid. They are concerned with calcium metabolism.

Adrenal glands

These are small paired glands beside each kidney and consist of two quite distinct parts. The outer part is the cortex, which produces a large number of fatty substances known as corticosteroids. The corticosteroids have three main functions: they control mineral and carbohydrate metabolism and reduce sensitivity and immunity reactions. Corticosteroids are widely used in human and veterinary medicine to assist the body's recovery, prevent over-reaction and allergies to infections and foreign substances. The inner part of the kidney – the medulla – produces adrenalin, the hormone of 'fright, flight and fight', i.e. it prepares the body to react to catastrophes and stress.

The pancreas

Much of the tissue of the pancreas is concerned with digestion and for this function the gland has a duct. However, within the gland are the Islets of Langerhan which act as an endocrine gland. They produce insulin which converts the glucose in the blood into glycogen – an insoluble carbohydrate which is stored as a reserve in the liver and muscles. Insulin and adrenalin act in an antagonistic way to produce a balance – insulin arranging the storage of potential energy and adrenalin making it available.

The pituitary gland

This small gland is situated at the base of the brain. The hormones produced by the pituitary gland control the development of the reproductive organs, the reproductive cycle, successful pregnancy, the development of the udder and the let-down of milk. The pituitary is responsible for initiating this activity but it also influences other endocrine organs, particularly the thyroid and adrenal cortex.

One hormone from the pituitary with little connection with the reproductive organs is the growth hormone – the rate of secretion during the growing period being largely responsible for the ultimate size of the individual.

The reproductive hormones of the pituitary

The follicle stimulating hormone (FSH)
Before puberty this helps growth of the reproductive organs in the male and female. After puberty FSH brings the ovarian follicle to maturity.

Luteinising hormone (LH)
LH causes the follicle to burst, releasing the ovum. It then provides the stimulus for the production of the corpus luteum in the crater resulting from the burst follicle. The follicular fluid and the corpus luteum produce further hormones. In the male, FSH is responsible for the development of sperm and LH stimulates the growth of the supporting tissue in the testicles where the sperm are produced.

Oxytocin
Oxytocin is a hormone from the pituitary which has a number of effects. It acts rapidly, particularly on the udder tissue, causing a let-down of milk into the cistern above the teat. The secretion is influenced by any action or noise associated with the process; for example, the noise of the piglets or butting of the udder, or in cows any action associated with the normal milking routine.

The reproductive organ hormones

Oestrogen

This hormone causes oestrus. The principal formation is in the follicular fluid of the ovary. The hormone is, in fact, produced in small quantities early in life, even in fetal life and results in the female conformation. When a follicle becomes large the increased production of oestrogen has an effect on the uterus and results in the behaviour known as oestrus or heat. When a follicle bursts the oestrogen is lost but the corpus luteum which replaces it secretes progesterone which causes a quiescent state in the muscles of the uterine wall and at the same time stimulates production of nutriment from the uterine wall and other activities in preparation of the embryo. If conception takes place the corpus luteum persists and progesterone continues to act as a stimulus to enlargement of the uterus and also leads to an increase in milk-secreting tissue in the udder.

Progesterone

Progesterone has an antagonistic effect on the pituitary gland, tending to suppress the production of FSH and LH so that during pregnancy ovarian follicles remain quiescent and oestrus does not occur, a rule with only the rarest exceptions. Pregnancy can usually be ended if the corpus luteum is squeezed off the ovary of the cow by manipulation through the wall of the rectum.

When conception does not take place the corpus luteum develops only for about half of the oestrus cycle and then regresses. Progesterone is then secreted in ever-decreasing amounts, the pituitary becomes more active and one or more follicles enlarge as oestrus occurs. Figure 2.14 illustrates the oestrous cycle of the sow.

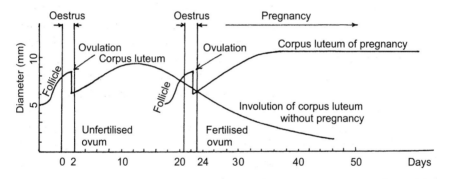

Fig. 2.14   The oestrous cycle of the sow (after Corner). Note the enlargement of the follicle and the regression of the corpus luteum if fertilisation does not occur. If the follicle is fertilised, the corpus luteum enlarges and persists during pregnancy.

Testosterone

Testosterone is produced in the testicles and brings about male characteristics and the development of the secondary male organs such as the prostate gland.

Prostaglandins

Prostaglandins are important hormones produced by the reproductive organs of both sexes. Their main functions of practical interest are in female reproduction but many tissues have been found to contain prostaglandins. Prostaglandins are frequently used in veterinary medicine to induce parturition and also to stimulate oestrus, recreating their normal functions in the body.

The development of the fetus

The fetus begins as a fertilised ovum which then continually divides. The embryo, as it is now called, comes to reside in a horn of the uterus where further nutriment is derived from the secretions of the glands in the uterine wall. The first differentiation is into three tissue layers which develop as follows.

The *ectoderm* gives rise to the skin and central nervous system, the *endoderm* gives rise to the alimentary canal and the *mesoderm* to the organs and tissues in between. At an early stage the layers fold over as if to form a cylinder and the ectoderm, as its name implies, becomes continuous on the outside, except for the area of the umbilicus whence the foetal membranes are rapidly formed. The membranes are initially a fluid-containing sac which grows up over the top of the fetus from each end. When the two ends meet fusion occurs in such a way as to produce two separate membranes around the fetus, each containing liquid. Thereafter the fetus is suspended in this double-skinned, fluid-filled container, which protects it from buffeting. The two membranes are together known as the placenta, at parturition they become the afterbirth. The different tissues and organs of the fetus develop with rapidly.

As the female approaches the end of her pregnancy the udder enlarges and milk will begin to be secreted. The vulva becomes enlarged and up to 48 hours before parturition the sacrosciatic ligament will slacken. The animal, if free, will tend to draw away alone from her fellows and will often cease to feed. Sows will make nests if given the opportunity. Labour pains mark the beginning of parturition – these being caused by the contraction of the uterine muscles. Labour pains come in spasms, the interval between them becoming less and less as parturition progresses. Sows grunt, sheep bleat and cows bellow in response to these pains.

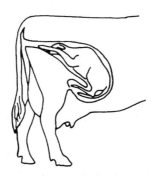

Fig. 2.15 Normal position of calf in the uterus before delivery.

The cervix must open and the vagina dilate. Under the pressure of the uterine muscles, the fluid-filled placenta enters the cervical canal. This placental sac is known as the water-bag, it tends to go through the vagina and then extends outside the vulva. The bag usually bursts to be followed by the birth of the young. After the young are born the afterbirth is expelled.

Figure 2.15 shows the normal position of a calf before delivery, but there may be abnormalities in parturition, such as the presentation being backwards or the limbs being retracted or the head being retained in a sideways position. In general, difficult malpresentations should be dealt with by the veterinary surgeon.

Chapter 3

Disease, Immunity and Welfare

Organisms causing infections

A substantial number of microorganisms cause disease in livestock and it is useful to classify these (Table 3.1).

The smallest organisms causing disease are the viruses, which are below 300 mμ in size. Many viruses are even smaller than this; for example, the foot-and-mouth disease viruses are 10–27 mμ (1μ = 0.001 mm and 1 mμ = 0.000001 mm). Viruses cannot usually be seen under the ordinary

Table 3.1 A summary of the living organisms causing disease.

Organism	Size range	Main characteristics
Viruses	From 10 mμ (0.00001 mm) to 300 mμ	The smallest group of pathogenic organisms. Can only multiply in living cells. Often very contagious. Quite vulnerable to destruction outside the body.
Bacteria	From 0.1 μ (0.0001 mm)	Relatively large. Great variety of size and shape. Can multiply and grow outside animal cells. Can form spores to resist destruction for many years. Contagious but less so than viruses.
Mycoplasma	0.25–0.5 μ	Resemble large viruses but they can multiply outside animal cells like bacteria. Moderately contagious in nature.
Rickettsia	0.25–0.4 μ	Similar in size to mycoplasma but only multiply in cells like viruses.
Fungi	0.1 μ–5 mm	Rapid multiplication under warm, damp conditions. Easy survival. Quite resistant to disinfection.
Parasites	1 μ–300 mm	From animal kingdom. Live whole or part of their lives on or within animals. Life cycles often complex with secondary hosts. Range from single-cell protozoa, such as coccidia, to parasites of ever increasing size and complexity, e.g. helminths, lice, flies and ticks.

microscope but can be photographed by the electron microscope. They are simple organisms that can only multiply within living cells, and this property distinguishes them from bacteria. Viruses are classified into a substantial number of different groups, e.g. reoviruses, adenoviruses and herpesviruses.

Compared with viruses bacteria are relatively large organisms and can multiply and grow outside living tissues. In size, for example, cocci (round) bacteria measure 0.8–1.2 µ, rods (bacilli) are 0.2–2 µ and the spiral-shaped spirella grow up to 50 µ; they are visible under the ordinary microscope. Many types, once outside the animal body, may sporulate to form a protective coat so that they can live for many years in buildings, soil or elsewhere yet still be capable of infecting animal life; for example, the spores of anthrax and clostridium can live for 20 years or more under favourable circumstances.

Mycoplasma are smaller organisms than bacteria, being about 0.25–0.5 µ (or 250–500 mµ). They are rather like oversized viruses but, unlike viruses, they can be cultured on artificial media.

Rickettsia are somewhat smaller than mycoplasma, being 0.256–0.4 µ, but they cannot be grown in ordinary culture media and will only multiply intracellularly, like viruses.

Varieties of fungi (moulds and yeasts), which are much larger than bacteria, cause disease in both humans and animals.

There are also many simple organisms from the animal kingdom, known as parasites, that cause disease in farm livestock. These range from the single-cell protozoa, such as the coccidial parasite, to parasites of ever increasing size and complexity, culminating in such relatively complicated organisms as the roundworms (helminths), lice, flies and ticks.

There are also other living and contagious pathogenic organisms which have yet to be fully identified, such as those which cause scrapie in sheep or bovine spongiform encephalopathy in cattle and other ungulates. Known as prions, these disease-causing agents are still not fully elucidated, despite years of research.

Organisms from these groups are the main cause of infectious disease in farm livestock. The only other agents causing disease and which are not infectious are the metabolic diseases, poisons, deficiencies, excesses and injuries, examples of which are found throughout the book.

Immunity

In our understanding of the mechanism of disease control it is essential to know the principles of the animal's immunological disease control system and the way in which we make use of such products as vaccines and anti–sera to boost it as necessary. This is best understood by studying the cycle of events in any animal's life.

When an animal is born it is relatively free of disease organisms but it has what is known as *passive immunity*, which it receives from the mother whilst still *in utero*. If the mother has been vaccinated against a disease or has had an experience of the actual disease, then her immunological system will produce the antibodies that are capable of resisting the disease. These antibodies circulate in the blood and will also be transferred to the fetus. The antibodies themselves are effective only for about 2–3 weeks before they disappear.

The young animal can produce only its own antibodies and thus develop what is known as *active immunity* if it has experienced the disease organisms in question, or has been vaccinated against them. It should be stressed that an animal will have some passive immunity only to those particular infections experienced by the mother. These may be quite limited and 'local'. This is a good argument for rearing an animal in the environment in which it is conceived and born and a good reason for not transporting young animals too early in life, before they have greater ability to resist a 'foreign' disease challenge. Passive immunity in mammals is fortified immediately after birth by the young drawing the first milk (or colostrum) from the dam. Colostrum is especially rich in antibodies and also nutrients and laxatives.

As the passive immunity the young animal receives from its mother wanes, it may be replaced by an active immunity if the young animal is vaccinated or has some exposure to organisms that can cause disease. Under practical conditions the aim is to make sure that any natural challenge of potentially pathogenic organisms is mild or gradual, not massive and over-whelming.

Sometimes it is perfectly satisfactory to allow the animals to receive a 'natural' challenge from the environment, but this is at best inexact and at worst ineffective. Thus, various methods of induced immunity are given, either *passive* or *active* (Fig. 3.1). The passive immunity is induced by injecting into the animal hyper-immune antiserum prepared from the serum of animals which have experienced the actual infection and which have recovered. This serum may be used for treatment of the disease and for passive immunity but has only a transitory effect lasting about 3 weeks, similar to the natural immunity received by the young animal from its mother.

For an active immunity, vaccines are used. A vaccine is a way of activating the body's defence mechanism by challenging it with pathogenic organisms modified so that they are just active enough to produce an immunity but not the disease itself. The modification can be done in many ways: by adding

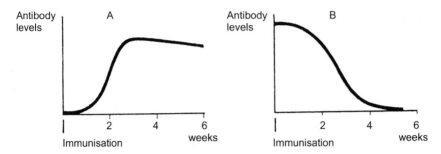

Fig. 3.1   Immunity. The curves in the diagrams represent antibody levels produced by active and passive immunisation. (A) shows the gradual development of
antibodies after active immunisation, as with a vaccine. (B) shows the immediate but
short-lived protection from passive immunity, as with hyperimmune serum.

chemicals, by growth of the organism in special media or livestock of a
different species, or by irradiation. Sometimes no modification is required as
an organism can be used which is sufficiently closely related to induce
immunity but not disease.

The production of vaccines is a very sophisticated process but can
induce an enormously efficient protection for the animal. Vaccines must be
used by skilled hands at the right time in the correct dose and repeated as
necessary since the immunities developed vary in their longevity according
to the infection. It should be borne in mind that when a vaccine is given
the immunity takes time to develop – usually about 3 weeks – so it may be
necessary to protect an animal during that time by antisera, antibiotics or
simply by isolation. Some vaccines are of live organisms, others are dead.
In general the live vaccine may give a stronger immunity more quickly but
it is not necessarily any longer lasting and it may induce more reaction.
Dead vaccines in an oil or other special base are very effective for long-
term immunities and are increasingly widely used. It should be emphasised
that when a vaccine is administered to an animal it causes a degree of illness
and during the period of immunological development the animal is
experiencing stress and is *more* susceptible to infection than at other times.
Thus it is necessary to practise even better management at the time of
vaccination. Very often this factor is not appreciated and a failure that is
unjustifiably ascribed to the vaccine is essentially due to mismanagement of
the animals.

Increasingly sophisticated techniques are being developed for the
production of vaccines which promise even better protection. In the future
it is anticipated that the prevention of disease in animals will be based on
greatly improved techniques of vaccination together with perfection in
methods of hygiene.

Veterinary medicines

Vaccines and sera are used to protect or treat animals for specific diseases. They should be used wherever they can in the prevention of infections; however, in many cases no serum or vaccine exists and we must deal with illness using one or many of a wide choice of medicines. Also, many of the disease conditions we are dealing with are caused by a number of different organisms. Often these are primary viral agents and secondary bacterial ones and, indeed, their identity may not be known for certain. Frequently the urgent need for treatment demands that a medicine is used before laboratory examinations have elucidated the cause, and we must rely on the clinical skill of the veterinarian to judge the correct medicine to use. When the results of the tests are known, an appropriate change in treatment may be indicated.

Medicines can be given to have an almost immediate action. One administration may have an effect for only a few hours or in some cases for a few days but usually, in order to keep the levels up within the bloodstream of the animal, there must be a constant boosting of levels. It cannot be emphasised too strongly that the full course of treatment prescribed should be completed and levels maintained correctly or the benefits may be lost and medicine-resistant organisms produced; this possibility is one of the worst outcomes of the use of medicines. Care must also be taken in the agricultural use of medicines to observe certain conditions of use. For example, with many medicines a compulsory withdrawal period is required before animals can be sent for slaughter, varying from about 5 to 10 days, and milk from cows being treated for mastitis must also not be mixed with normal milk for specified periods. Ignorance of the correct procedure can be disastrous.

The majority of medicines used for the prevention and treatment of disease are *chemotherapeutics* – the term implying the use of chemicals that have either been synthesised (such as the sulphonamides) or produced by the action of living organisms (antibiotics). Modern research is continually producing new medicines and great credit is due to the active research in this field which is responsible for the vast armoury of safe materials for use in livestock husbandry.

The routes by which medicines are given vary from injection by the intravenous, intramuscular or subcutaneous routes to oral dosing and incorporation in feed or drinking water. With so many medicines available and the routes and methods of administration being so variable it is perhaps inevitable that careless and abusive use occurs. One cannot do more than emphasise that the prescription of medicines requires a high degree of skill and their administration an abundance of diligence and competence.

Probiotics

Probiotics may be defined as living microorganisms which when fed to animals assist in the establishment of an intestinal population which is beneficial to the animal and antagonistic to harmful (pathogenic) microbes. Available probiotic cultures consist of specific counts of bacteria maintained in a dry form for storage purposes, and produce an optimal response within a specified dose range. Their usage is increasing as our understanding of their value is further elucidated.

Approved probiotics

Extensive investigation and research has been carried out on those probiotics approved for use and their benefits may be summarised as follows:

(1)   Probiotics can promote growth and productivity in livestock in a natural way
(2)   Probiotics may protect against *Salmonella* infections, including the worst types such as *S. enteritidis* and *S. typhimurium*
(3)   They can protect against toxins produced by harmful forms of *E. coli*
(4)   Probiotics stimulate immunity to infections by boosting interferon production, immunoglobulin concentration and macrophage activity
(5)   Probiotics suppress clostridial infections which are often associated with intensive livestock production
(6)   Probiotics have also been shown to be antagonistic to many other harmful bacteria, such as *Klebsiella, Proteus* and *Campylobacter*
(7)   There is research evidence that probiotics are active against the development of cancers in animals

Tender loving care

Under perfectly normal modern methods of livestock husbandry, whether extensive or intensive, and however good they may be, there will always be stressful periods and inevitable disease challenges. The best way of enabling animals to meet these pressures is to boost their own natural resistance. Probiotics can achieve this by helping the animal complete and supplement its internal microflora. Widespread evidence has shown that the use of probiotics can promote the growth and productivity of livestock and act as a protection against infections such as *Salmonella* and *Campylobacter*.

There are, however, some vital cautionary points to emphasise. The chosen probiotic should contain a number of species so that a wide spectrum of activity is ensured. Also, the user should choose the product carefully on this basis and on the assurance and advice of the probiotic producer. Probiotics are living products and need to be handled with care.

The method of inclusion and administration, whether in the drinking water or in the feed, and the dosage to be applied require a combination of expert advice from the manufacturer or adviser and care by the owner of the livestock. The products need to be treated like the livestock – with tender loving care.

Growth promoters

For many years the livestock industry has made use of antibiotics and other substances which, when incorporated in very small amounts in the ration, tend to increase the growth rate of livestock and improve food conversion efficiency. In the early days of use of these materials, the same antibiotics were used for growth promotion as for the treatment of disease. Since medicines as growth promoters are used at a much lower level than for therapeutic use, incorporating antibiotics at a low level into the feed is disastrous since medicine-resistant organisms will soon emerge and not only will the antibiotics no longer be of use as growth promoters but they will also have lost their value for therapeutic purposes. Because of this there is now a clear separation, legally enforced, between the use of antibiotics for these two purposes. Those antibiotics that are used as growth promoters (e.g. zinc bacitracin, Flavomycin and Virginiamycin) have no other use and are not used for any therapeutic purposes. Furthermore, the therapeutic antibiotics are used only for prevention and treatment of disease and are available only on veterinary prescription to be used under the control of the veterinary surgeon.

This problem of resistance is not the only one caused by feeding growth-promoting antibiotics to livestock. These substances have their greatest effect when the hygiene or husbandry system is less than ideal. Under really good management practices they may do little good at all. Thus growth-promoting antibiotics tend to 'mask' bad husbandry and this is potentially dangerous since such an effect will not last for ever, unlike the bad practices, which will tend to have a cumulative effect on results. It may sometimes be argued that the use of growth promoters is to be deprecated altogether but I disagree: it must always be borne in mind that it is impossible, under commercial conditions, for everything always to be ideal. Better, therefore, to use growth promotors as an aid but not to rely on them absolutely.

There is still no absolute certainty as to the means by which growth-promoting antibiotics exert their effects, but it seems most likely they are due to their favourable action on the balance of bacteria in the intestines:

reducing the harmful ones and promoting the beneficial ones and thereby increasing the efficiency of food utilisation and production.

The importance of disinfection

Almost all livestock and even those kept outdoors are now housed much more intensively than before. This involves not only stocking animals more densely but also an increased size of units and more efficient use of building or grazing space. It is rare for a livestock pen to be without stock; if there is a break between batches then it is usually a short-lived one. In the days before the use of antibiotic therapy, intensive methods tended to collapse under the burden of disease, now they are again under threat because an increasing number of disease-producing organisms are resistant to medicines and the cost of almost continuous antibiotic therapy is becoming an economically damaging and unacceptable burden to the stock keeper.

It is now appreciated that there is one viable alternative to the increasing cost of therapy which is to institute a very efficient programme of cleaning and disinfection of the buildings. Let us be quite clear, however: disinfection needs to be done in a carefully organised way and must not be, as so often is the case, an application of some disinfectant chosen at random in the hope that it will kill the pathogens. First, it is imperative – at least with young livestock – to plan the enterprise in such a way that a building or even a site is totally depopulated of stock before the cleaning and disinfection takes place. This is necessary because the live animal – and it might literally be only one – is potentially a much greater reservoir of infection than the building itself. The disinfection process in sequence is shown in Table 3.2.

There must be a careful consideration of the different requirements of young and old housed animals. Young animals are born with only a limited immunity to infection and this can very quickly wane. It is usually essential that the young animal receives a very limited exposure to disease in the first few weeks of life particularly and this is best achieved if it is born in very clean quarters. Thus in limiting the challenge of disease it is essential to have buildings of small size, thereby reducing the number of animals, and only animals of one age group, if possible, as these are more likely to have the same levels of immunity and they can build up this immunity together without competition.

With much older animals and, in particular, the adult, the position may be totally different. The animals may have a considerable degree of immunity to local pathogens so that there is no merit to giving them totally clean buildings. What may be required here is a rather different standard of underlying good hygiene to prevent gross infection and contamination.

Table 3.2 The disinfection process in sequence.

(1) Empty the pen and preferably the house and site of all livestock
(2) Clean out all 'organic matter' – dung, bedding, old feed, any other material that could contain pathogenic microorganisms – and remove totally from the area of the building
(3) Remove all portable equipment for cleaning and disinfecting outside the building
(4) Wash down with heavy-duty detergent–steriliser. Use a power washer wherever possible
(5) Apply a disinfection or disinfectants appropriate to the type of infections being dealt with. Usually required is a mixture active against viruses, bacteria, parasites and insects which may carry infection from one batch of livestock to another. Specialist advice is often required on the choice of the correct disinfectant.
(6) Wherever possible fumigate or spray with a disinfectant after the equipment and litter have been reassembled
(7) Dry out between each of the disinfectant applications
(8) Always complete one process throughout the site before starting the next
(9) The area in close proximity to the buildings requires an equal attention to its hygiene at the end of each crop

Practical hygiene

How does one go about setting up the hygienic programme in practice? First of all there will probably be some differences in the construction of the building. With animals which are very young, or in poultry the hatchery and incubator, the aim is almost total sterilisation. This can be achieved only by raising the standard of construction of the surfaces, which must be both smooth and impervious so that they can be thoroughly cleaned (Fig. 3.2).

With knowledge of the diseases that are causing risk to the animals, a suitable range of disinfectants can be chosen. Such a programme of disinfectants may well include the application of disinfectants *and* fumigants. Disinfection is likely to involve the elimination of viruses, bacteria, fungi and parasites. With the housing of adults, however, the position is rather different. Because the disease risk is less, the construction of the buildings may not be to such a high standard; for example, timber construction may be widespread and floors may be of earth or chalk rather than impervious concrete. Furthermore, the range of infections under consideration may be less comprehensive – bacterial agents possibly being the worst that have to be dealt with – but the animal may already have a fairly high degree of immunity, for example, to viruses. Thus it can be said that whilst measures may not be so complicated, it is still very important to choose the right agents and apply them in the correct way (Figs 3.3–3.4).

The safety of medicines

There are very demanding regulations covering the supply of all medicinal products, including vaccines, in the animal health field. Before any such

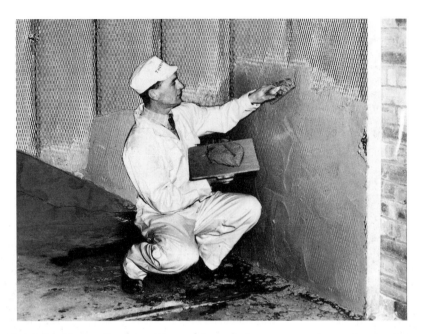

Fig. 3.2 The application of a smooth rendering on an under-surface insulation layer ensures cleanliness, warmth and less likelihood of condensation.

product can be made available for livestock it must be tested for safety, quality and efficacy. In addition, when it is given to any animal that can enter the human food chain – or produce a product, such as milk or eggs, that enters the food chain – the regulatory authorities must be satisfied that there are no harmful residues of the medicines in the food product. The regulations may therefore forbid the use of certain medicines to any animal that is used for food, or a 'withdrawal' period may be specified in which there is a safe gap between the use of the product and the entry of the animal or its products into the food chain. There is sound practical analytical evidence that food is safe in this respect; furthermore, many products which were once used, such as hormones and stimulants based on arsenicals, are now totally banned for any use at all. Many of the 'scares' over food safety generated by lobby groups and enlarged by the media are not justified in this instance and there is no evidence that any harm has been done to humans.

Signs of health and disease

The early recognition of illness is particularly vital in the intensive unit because the risk of anything that is contagious spreading is very great. Early recognition increases the opportunity for successful treatment, enables the

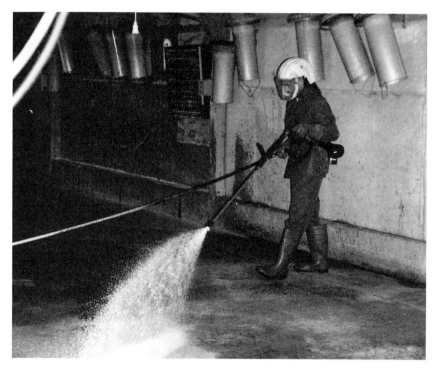

Fig. 3.3 For disinfection to be effective it must be preceded by proper cleansing.

affected stock to be isolated and speeds any laboratory diagnostic work. It also helps in the good welfare of the animals since sick animals are often maltreated by their neighbours. All in all, early recognition of ill health will generally reduce losses to a minimum, and thus makes sound economic sense.

There are certain signs to look for which may indicate illness; these are discussed in the following sections.

Feeding

One of the earliest and surest signs of illness is a lack of interest in feed (anorexia) or a capricious appetite, although occasionally it is the feed itself which is at fault and requires investigation.

Separation from the group

Sick animals will usually separate from the healthy and hide in a corner or bury themselves in bedding, if available and if there is the space to do it.

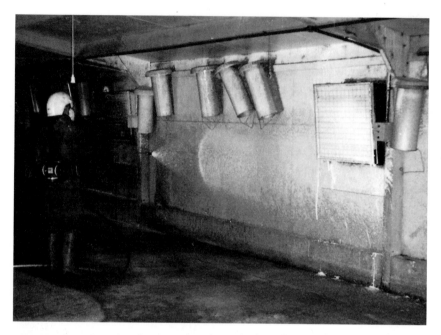

Fig. 3.4   Modern disinfectant solution applied to clean surfaces, even if porous, can be effective if allowed sufficient time to act.

Excreta

This may be 'abnormal'. Sick animals often have scour (diarrhoea) or, more usually in the earliest stages of disease, they will be constipated, especially if there is a fever. In other circumstances the faeces may contain blood (dysentery) or may be of abnormal colour (which sometimes happens in cases of poisoning, for example, but is occasionally diagnostic in nature with certain infections).

Urine

This may show abnormalities, such as the presence of blood, or may be cloudy or yellow (jaundiced). Normal urine is rather pale and straw-coloured.

Posture

Sick animals may find it impossible to rise, may hold themselves uncomfortably, or may be lame. The nature of the abnormality of posture may indicate the organ which is affected.

Appearance

Sick animals will often have a droopy head, with dull eyes and dry muzzle and possibly a discharge from the nose and watery or catarrhal eyes. All the mucous membranes may be discoloured.

Skin and coat

A healthy coat is clean and glossy. Abnormal coats may be 'hidebound', which is when hydration makes it difficult to move the skin over the underlying tissues. Sick animals may have bald, scurfy, 'lousy', mangy or scabby skin and the animals may scratch or rub. The skin, coat and feathers are very good indicators of disease.

Coughing

Most abnormalities of the respiratory system produce coughing in animals and the nature of the cough will often be diagnostic of certain conditions.

Pain

The presence of pain shows in a number of ways: grunts, groans, grinding of the teeth, squealing or crying, arching of the back.

Temperature

An abnormally high temperature usually indicates an infection; an abnormally low one may be due to a metabolic defect, a poisoning or simply the later or terminal stages of an infection. Normal temperatures and respirations are set out in Table 3.3.

Table 3.3 Normal temperatures and respiration rates.

| | Temperature | | Respirations |
	(°C)	(°F)	per minute
Cattle	38.7	101.5	12–20
Sheep	39.4	103.0	12–30
Pig	39.2	102.5	10–18
Fowl	41.5	106.5	12–28

Respirations tend to be accelerated by infectious diseases and slowed by others, although the nature of the breathing will also be vastly affected and may change from deep to shallow on the occurrence of illness.

Pulse rates

These are normally only studied by the veterinarian, but the normal rates are set out in Table 3.4.

Table 3.4   Normal pulse rates.

	Pulse rate per minute
Cattle	45–50
Sheep	70–90
Pig	70–80
Fowl	130–140

Animal welfare and animal health

Disquiet exists over the humanity of some of the more modern and intensive methods of rearing livestock. Certain practices have come under critical attack from welfare groups, especially keeping chickens in battery cages, housing calves in 'crates' for the production of veal and keeping sows closely tethered in stalls during pregnancy. In the UK it is now illegal to rear calves in 'crates' and from 1999 it will be illegal to keep sows tethered or in individual stalls without the ability to turn around. Having been personally involved in this controversy since it started and looking back on 40 years' involvement in the management of intensive livestock, I am convinced that the dispute has been beneficial since it has thrown a very sharp light on methods and forced everyone involved to think carefully about what they are doing. It is now leading rather belatedly to active research and investigation which may answer some of our doubts. Table 3.5 summarises the essentials of livestock welfare.

Animal welfare is also very pertinent to the question of health since there is no dispute that one of the essential criteria for the provision of good welfare is the maintenance of health in the animals. It has also become apparent from recent activities in the research field that the eventual goal of establishing what constitutes good welfare in a scientific way is going to be very difficult indeed, if not impossible. Thus we shall have to continue to rely, at least in the foreseeable future, on the overall knowledge, expertise and even instinct of the people concerned with the management and care of the animals, these being the farmers, stockmen, and husbandry and veterinary advisers. It is essential to keep in the forefront of one's mind the overriding importance of welfare and humanity to animals on all occasions. Anyone who has closely observed sick animals can understand what constitutes 'misery' in the animal kingdom and contrast this with the alert and buoyant appearance of an animal in good health.

Table 3.5 The essentials for welfare.

(1) Enough space should be provided for the animals to move around freely – to stretch their limbs or wings, to turn around and groom or preen themselves

(2) All surfaces, especially flooring, must be comfortable and unlikely to cause injury (Fig. 3.5)

(3) A suitable 'micro-climate' should be provided, that is, appropriate ambient temperature, humidity, air movement and ventilation

(4) All measures must be taken to ensure healthy stock

(5) A balanced ration should be available in sufficient quantity and of a suitable consistency for the animals' digestive system. Clean water or another appropriate liquid should always be accessible

(6) Groups of animals should be evenly matched. If animals are kept individually they should be within sight of others

(7) All sick animals and 'bullies' must be removed and isolated from healthy stock

(8) There should be adequate provision to cope with emergencies, such as fire and electrical or mechanical failures

(9) Wherever possible bedding should be provided, such as clean straw or wood shavings

(10) Mutilations on animals, such as beak trimming of birds or de-tailing of pigs, should not be undertaken except under exceptional circumstances when more suffering might result if it were *not* done. Alternative husbandry systems which do not require mutilations should be considered

(11) Lighting should be generous for the management of the animals and adequate at all other times

(12) Regulations regarding the transport of livestock should be followed (Fig. 3.6)

A feature of this controversial field which has been particularly beneficial is the way in which it has forced us to enquire whether it is necessary to house animals using methods which involve an abnormal degree of restriction on their movement. There has been a search for alternatives which has been fruitful insofar as it appears to indicate that there may be less need for the extremes of intensification that have been alleged and indeed it may be economically preferable to have systems which are more in harmony with the overall agricultural scene.

Very large and intensive livestock enterprises have often been unsuccessful and even disastrous for three principal reasons. First, the management of large numbers of *living beings* is not easily organised on a large scale. Stockmanship is partly science and partly art, and art must rely heavily on the individual. If only one small item goes wrong or is overlooked it can lead to a very serious chain of events on a large scale.

The second reason is that disease is much more likely to have a serious deleterious effect in a large unit, either in sub-clinical or clinical forms. The failure of many units can be ascribed to their inability to control disease so that the economic viability of the unit has been totally destroyed (see Chapter 1).

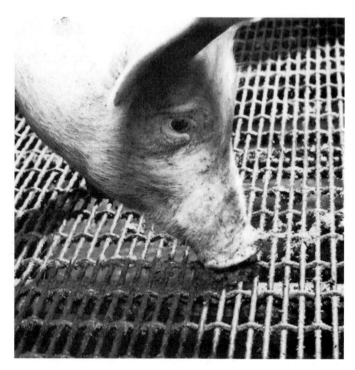

Fig. 3.5   Perforated pig flooring – a form of mesh which is self-cleaning but with risks of disease.

The third reason is the heavy cost of buying in or bringing in fodder and moving out the muck in such enterprises. It is common for the highly intensive unit to be totally dependent on food from outside the farm or the locality and to be faced with great difficulty in disposing of all the waste products. In smaller units the crops can be used to feed the livestock and the 'muck' they generate is of great value to the land; energy is conserved and this is agriculture of a totally balanced sort.

It may also be stated that the welfare standards that are gradually emerging across the world are based on evidence which, as far as is possible, is not in conflict with economics. For example, if animals are housed at concentrations and intensities above those advised, it is likely that their productivity will fall. This is particularly so when it comes to stocking density and its relationship to growth, production and the efficiency of food utilisation. Good welfare standards can be used, therefore, as a husbandry standard with some confidence.

The key to good welfare is a high standard of stockmanship and if this is to function then good facilities must be provided for the stockman; many

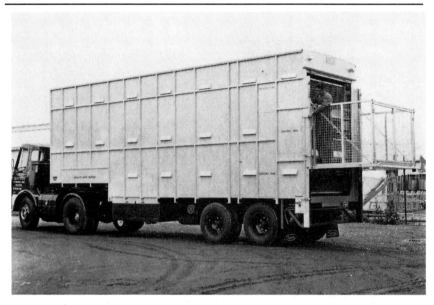

Fig. 3.6 This livestock transporter reduces the stress on the stock by its mechanical hoist and powered ventilation.

systems that have been developed in recent years completely ignore this. The essentials are as follows:

- ❑ Plenty of room for the stockman to *see* the stock whenever he needs to
- ❑ Good lighting and no undue saving on passage space
- ❑ Facilities for the isolation of sick stock
- ❑ Easy access by the stockman to the pen and, above all, a very high standard of handling facilities so that it is easy to medicate or treat the animals in any way necessary.

Disease legislation

In Great Britain, under the Diseases of Animals Act, there are a substantial number of orders relating essentially to the State's interest in animal disease control. These regulations cover a wide spectrum of activity. For example, they deal with the importation of animals and animal by-products, the movement of animals, the inspection of livestock and vehicles, and allow for the Ministry of Agriculture to institute a large number of orders relating essentially to specific diseases.

Under the Diseases of Animals Act certain specified diseases are designated notifiable; those of current importance are:

- ❑ Anthrax
- ❑ Bovine spongiform encephalopathy
- ❑ Foot and mouth disease
- ❑ Fowl pest
- ❑ Bovine tuberculosis
- ❑ Swine vesicular disease
- ❑ Aujeszky's disease
- ❑ Enzootic bovine leucosis
- ❑ Rabies
- ❑ Salmonellosis

There are also others, such as swine fever, which could well occur again as they are widespread not far from these shores.

The most important feature about the notifiable disease is that the owner or person in charge of an animal suspected to be affected by a notifiable disease must immediately report his suspicion to a police officer or an Inspector of the Ministry of Agriculture. Once the owner has notified the inspector or the police, steps will be taken to diagnose the condition and measures may be taken to isolate the premises and treat, vaccinate or slaughter the stock. Different diseases require different responses and these are dealt with later in the book in the discussions of the respective diseases. Also, under the Zoonoses Order, the presence of conditions such as salmonellosis and brucellosis, which infect both animals and man, must be notified.

Chapter 4

Diseases of Animals Communicable to Man: The Zoonoses

Until recently the general public apparently gave little attention to zoonoses, those diseases of animals which could pass to man. Now it is a different story and the consumer is constantly bombarded with information about the dangers of eating infected animal products. In addition the scares have extended to the perceived risks from eating products derived from animals which have been receiving unwise or uncontrolled, excessive doses of antibiotics and other medicines and 'growth promoters' of various kinds, including hormones.

In truth the media have had a field day. The present era of food scares effectively started with the statement from the former Junior Minister for Agriculture, Edwina Currie, in 1988 that alleged the majority of our poultry flock was contaminated with a particular form of salmonella which infected eggs and was capable of causing serious enteritis and even generalised disease in the human subject. Subsequent events, which will be dealt with later, proved this to be a grossly exaggerated statement. More recently, the great 'mad cow disease' scare has emerged. 'Mad cow disease' is a degenerative disease of cattle which is known as bovine spongiform encephalopathy, or BSE for short. This, it is claimed, is indistinguishable from an incurable disease of man known as Creutzfeldt-Jakob disease or CJD and it has been suggested, though without any conclusive proof, that BSE-infected cattle products could infect man to cause CJD. Other diseases of animals that may also infect man include tuberculosis, campylobacter, meningitis, listeriosis and *Escherichia coli* enteritis.

It is often alleged that zoonotic diseases have increased in their incidence. This may not be the case, instead it could be that the efficiency of recording and diagnosing the diseases could have improved. Diagnostic methods certainly have advanced immensely in recent years. It is also likely that patients are more easily persuaded to seek professional advice when suffering from an ailment; hence statistics can distort the evidence quite seriously.

I believe, from studying all the evidence, that the overall danger to the human consumer is small and getting smaller all the time. The media seize upon a few figures and exaggerate them out of all proportion. The fact that pathogenic organisms are found does not mean that they are a new feature; examples will show the evidence for this. *Salmonella enteritidis* and *S. typhimurium* infections were prevalent in broiler breeders and could thereby give rise to infection in broilers. Very great efforts have been made in the last few years to attempt a complete eradication of these two most pathogenic sources of salmonella from poultry. In fact these endeavours have gone well: *S. enteritidis* and *S. typhimurium* have both decreased markedly and eventual freedom from these agents should not be difficult. It can be seen from Fig. 4.1 that the incidence has decreased very steadily as it has also in animal feed, where recovery is now rare. There have also been further developments in vaccinal protection which enable the industry to foresee a complete elimination of pathogenic salmonella within the next year or two.

We can see the same state of affairs with anthrax, a disease which was once quite common as a cause of sudden death in cattle and of illness in pigs. It can be seen from Table 4.1 that cases have so diminished that only ten cases have occurred in the last 5 years.

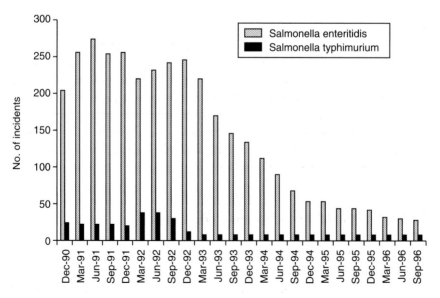

Fig. 4.1   Salmonella incidents in broiler breeders 1990–1996.

Table 4.1 Anthrax cases in Great Britain 1991–1995.

| Year | No. of investigations | Incidents | Deaths | | County |
			Animals	Number	
1991	9280	2	Cattle	1	Nottinghamshire
			Cattle	1	Strathclyde
1992	8516	2	Cattle	1	Derbyshire
			Cattle	1	Clwyd
1993	8662	2	Cattle	1	Derbyshire
			Cattle	4	Highlands
1994	8301	3	Cattle	3	Gloucestershire
			Cattle	1	Isle of Wight
			Cattle	1	Wiltshire
1995	7902	1	Cattle	1	Northamptonshire
1996	4521	1	Cattle	1	Northamptonshire

Scrapie cases in sheep – a disease strongly proposed as a forerunner to BSE – is also following a steady downward path (Fig. 4.2), with 209 cases on 112 premises reported in 1996.

The degree of challenge

It may also be emphasised that for infections to take place there has to be a certain strength of challenge, or, put another way, a certain number of the infecting organisms. This varies according to the nature of the infection and the susceptibility of the host, but one fact is clear: any measure taken to reduce the challenge is worthwhile, even if it is impossible to completely remove it altogether.

Table 4.2 shows how the dose of organisms that are required to produce an overt clinical disease in man may vary from some 100 in the case of *Listeria* disease to as many as 100 000 with *E. coli.*

The surveillance of residues

The UK has a National Sampling and Surveillance Scheme (NSS) in place which is designed to monitor whether veterinary medicines are passing into meat for human consumption. In 1996, 40 000 samples were taken and examined.

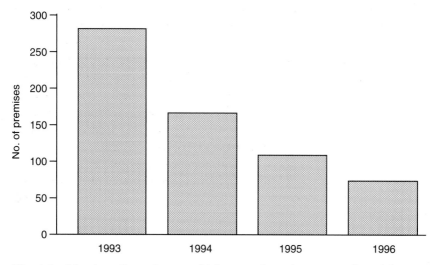

Fig. 4.2   Number of premises on which cases of scrapie were confirmed for years 1993–1996

Table 4.2   Bacterial food infections from poultry.

Bacteria	Main cause of infection	Infective dose	Major symptoms
Salmonella spp.	Temperature above 5°C in transport. Food insufficiently cooked	10 000	Enteritis and fever. Severe abdominal pain
Campylobacter jejuni	Dirty food handling. Food insufficiently cooked	100	Diarrhoea or dysentery fever, nausea. Severe abdominal pain
Listeria monocytogenes	Dirty food processing, production, handling and storage	100	Enteritis, fever, meningitis and abortion
Escherichia coli	Poor husbandry producing 'wet' litter or conditions. Poor techniques of handling birds from depletion to processing causing contamination of meat. Food insufficiently cooked or retained above 2°C for too long a period	100 000	Enteritis, dystentery haemolytic uraemia and kidney damage, severe abdominal pain

In fact the number of positives were very low. There was no evidence for the illegal use of hormones, synthetic steroids or clembuterol. A few low levels of antimicrobial compounds continue to occur, those present being identified as chlortetracycline, penicillin G, oxytetracycline, sulphadimidine, sulphadiazine and streptomycin. In 1996 six samples from sheep contained residues of penicillin G and only two samples from poultry were found to be positive. It is of significance that in spite of all the samples taken, there were no medicinal residues above the statutory levels in poultry meat. Thus the real risk to the human population is effectively nil and with increasing attention to enforcing the regulations the risk will continue to diminish, especially as we are moving towards using less medicinal treatment for disease and placing greater emphasis on hygiene and vaccination.

Statistics

There are lies, damn lies and statistics. Statistics on food poisoning and food safety can be very misleading and often misquoted. As emphasised earlier, the detection and diagnostic rate of food poisoning may have increased rather than the actual incidence. Furthermore, the causes have more to do with mass-catering, the popularity of fast food and bad handling. If the food is incorrectly handled it is inevitable that some bacteria will multiply and thereby enteritis or other disease may be caused in the human subject. A far greater understanding is required concerning the handling of foods after they have left the retailer.

From the very earliest stages of the salmonella and BSE sagas there has been a complete openness about the situation in the UK. However, because research and investigations into the conditions, especially BSE, are far from complete, the irresponsibility of the media and some scientists have attempted to present the worst possible scenario and the dangers have consequently become grossly exaggerated. Generally we do not see the same openness in other countries; the identical diseases generally occur but appear to be hushed up. Having seen the position for myself – after prolonged visits to Italy and France – I know that this is so. Under European legislation there should be harmony both in the regulations and their administration governing the safety of food and the control of animal diseases, especially zoonoses. In practice this does not happen. The laws of a country may be sufficient but the enforcement remains in the hands of that country itself. Enforcement in some countries is poor or lacking altogether, whereas in our own country it is much more rigid, even bordering on the excessive, insensitive and often unnecessarily demanding.

Types of zoonotic disease

Bacterial infection

In Table 4.3 a list is given of the most important of the zoonotic diseases. Some of these diseases are traditionally well known and the risks appreciated. For example, sudden death in cattle may be due to anthrax; checks are invariably made if anthrax is suspected and it is easy to diagnose. Tetanus is caused by another spore-bearing bacterium, *Clostridia tetani*, which can infect the human subject. Both anthrax and tetanus can rapidly be fatal, although if care is taken with the proper disposal of carcasses, correct hygiene and vaccination, any real risk is completely removed. In addition, any person at risk can be protected effectively by vaccination. Infection of the human subject with these diseases by direct animal contamination is very rare indeed in the UK but there are much larger risks abroad due to climate, higher incidences of the diseases and poorer sanitation and hygiene. The situation is not very different with bacterial animal infections, such as tuberculosis, brucellosis, leptospirosis and salmonellosis.

Two more bacterial diseases which have hit the headlines in what may be termed 'media scares' have been the bacteria *Listeria* and *Campylobacter*; these are both organisms of a universal distribution, but with certain predilections for contamination. Listeriosis in the human subject may often be traced to cheese made from unpasteurised milk or vegetables, whereas contaminated meat appears to be the principal culprit so far as campylobacter is concerned. Whilst the former may be a risk to the pregnant woman and is implicated as a cause of abortion, campylobacter is blamed for many cases of gastroenteritis. Fairly mild and certainly less severe than salmonellosis, campylobacter is no real danger to those other than the very young or very old. Nevertheless, statistically it is blamed for more cases of 'food poisoning' than salmonella but the cases are sporadic and far less serious.

In fact none of these bacterial diseases really require additional measures over and above the ones which have been emphasised already. *Campylobacter* bacteria, of which there are many types, can be associated in particular with the drinking water system and for a long time it has been justifiably recommended that the drinking water supply to farm livestock that are supplying the human food chain should be treated with an appropriate sanitiser, such as chlorine dioxide. This of course will not only help to limit campylobacter, but will reduce the challenge from all other contagions which may pass through or be spread by the water system.

In recent years a newly diagnosed cause of food poisoning has been the bacteria *Escherichia coli* 0157–H7. An outbreak in Scotland in 1996 involved some 300 people and there were 17 deaths. The agent causing the epidemic

Table 4.3 Zoonoses.

Name of disease	Infective organism	Livestock infected	Geographical distribution	Principal means of spread to man
Bacterial diseases				
Anthrax	*Bacillus anthracis*	Warm-blooded animals	Universal, especially warm climates	Human infections usually via skin but may be inhaled or ingested. Spores in the soil or in animal products are very resistant to destruction
Brucellosis	*Brucella abortus* B. melitensis B. suis	Cattle Goats, sheep Pigs	Universal but has been eradicated in many areas	Direct contact with excretions or secretions, including milk of infected animals
Campylobacteriosis	*Campylobacter* spp.	Many animals	Universal. Incidence is vastly increasing	Most species or sub-species appear to be reasonably host-specific but cross-infection is possible, usually via faecal contamination of food
Clostridial disease	*Clostridium* spp.	Mammals, birds, fish	Universal	Infection from injuries via spores in soil is the chief hazard for man but food poisoning occurs
Erysipeloid (Erysipelas in animals other than man)	*Erysipelothrix rhusiopathiae*	Pigs, turkeys, pigeons, sea mammals, fish	Universal	Infection of wounds
Escherichia coli	*E. coli* 0157-H7	Most livestock including cattle, pigs, sheep and poultry	Universal	Consumption of raw or undercooked meat products and now milk
Leptospirosis	*Leptospira* spp. (many serotypes)	Domestic and wild animals, especially rodents	Universal	In man, by direct contact with an infected animal's urine or tissue (or aborted fetus), or from contaminated soil or water

Table 4.3 Continued

Name of disease	Infective organism	Livestock infected	Geographical distribution	Principal means of spread to man
Listeriosis	*Listeria* spp.	Numerous animals and birds	Universal	Food-borne from domestic animal products inefficiently cooked or prepared
Melioidosis	*Pseudomonas pseudomallei*	Rodents, sheep, goats, horses, pigs, non-human primates, kangaroos	Asia, Australia, East Indies, South America, USA	Soil or water contamination of wounds, ingestion, inhalation, not from animal to animal
Plague	*Yersinia pestis*	Rodents, cats, dogs, others	Western USA, Central and South America, South-east Asia, southern Africa	Fleas, contact with infected animals, inhalation
Psittacosis (ornithosis)	*Chlamydia psittaci*	Parakeets, pigeons, parrots, turkeys, ducks, geese, etc.	Universal	By inhaling dust from faeces or feathers
Rat bite fever	*Streptobacillus (Actinobacillus moniliformis) Spirillum minus*	Rodents	Universal	Bites of rodents, ingestion, wounds
Salmonellosis	*Salmonella* spp., over 2000 serotypes	Poultry, pigs, cattle, horses, dogs, cats and birds	Universal	Usually from ingestion of undercooked or recooked food contaminated with faeces, handling diseased animals
Tetanus	*Clostridium tetani*	Cattle, sheep, horses	Universal	Wound infected from soil, especially if contaminated with faeces

Disease	Organism	Hosts	Distribution	Transmission
Tuberculosis	*Mycobaterium bovis*	Cattle, non-human primates	Universal	Ingestion, inhalation
	M. tuberculosis	Monkeys and other non-human primates, rarely dogs, cats, other domestic animals	Universal	Exposure to animals infected with human tuberculosis
Yersiniosis	*Yersinia pseudotuberculosis* *Y. enterocolitica*	Animals and birds	Northern Hemisphere	Contaminated food or water

Fungal diseases

Many fungal diseases occur in man and other animals, but most are rare, and generally the result of environmental exposure rather than of cross-species contagion. Ringworm is a 'true zoonosis'

Disease	Organism	Hosts	Distribution	Transmission
Ringworm	*Microsporum* spp. *Trichophyton* spp.	Many mammals and birds	Universal	Direct contact with infected animals and fomites

Parasitic diseases

Protozoan diseases

Disease	Organism	Hosts	Distribution	Transmission
Sarcosporidiosis	*Sarcocystis* spp.	Pigs, cattle, sheep, ducks	Worldwide	Ingestion of meat
Toxoplasmosis	*Toxoplasma gondii*	Mammals (especially cats), birds	Worldwide	Ingestion of oocysts shed in faeces of infected cats and meat that contains cysts

Cestode (tapeworm) infections

Disease	Organism	Hosts	Distribution	Transmission
Beef tapeworm, Cysticerosis	*Taenia saginata*	Cattle, buffalo, giraffe, llama	Universal	Ingestion of 'measly' beef
Echinococcosis, Hydatid	*Echinococcus granulosus*	Cats, wild carnivores, sheep, cattle	Universal	Ingestion of eggs shed in faeces of carnivores
Pork tapeworm, Cysticercosis	*Taenia solium*	Pigs, others	Worldwide	Ingestion of 'measly' pork, autoinfection

Table 4.3 Continued

Name of disease	Infective organism	Livestock infected	Geographical distribution	Principal means of spread to man
Diseases caused or borne by arthropods				

It is not uncommon for persons handling animals infested with mites (usually *Sarcoptes* spp.) or fleas (e.g. from dogs or birds) to become infested, although usually the infestation on the abnormal host is short-lived. This can, however, lead to significant discomfort or, on occasion, to transmission of other diseases, e.g. plague. Rarely, screwworms or bot flies infest man. Various ticks infest man as well as other animals, and the consequences may be serious. Some ticks cause paralysis of their hosts (including man) via envenomisation. The greatest dangers lie not in the arthropod infestation itself, but in the diseases for which the arthropods may serve as vectors. Several encephalitides, hemorrhagic fevers, rickettsias, and protozoal blood parasites are transmitted by arthropods. Arthropod-borne bacterial diseases include Lyme disease, plague and tularemia.

Name of disease	Infective organism	Livestock infected	Geographical distribution	Principal means of spread to man
Viral diseases				
African green monkey disease	Marburg virus	African green monkey (*Cecopithecus aethiops*)	Central Africa	Contacted with infected tissues
Bovine spongiform encephalopathy (BSE)	Prion ('slow virus')	Cattle	Principally UK	Assumed by consumption of infected nervous tissue but not proven
Contagious ecthyma (Orf)	Parapoxvirus	Sheep, goats	Universal	Contact exposure
Cowpox	Poxvirus	Cattle	Universal	Contact exposure
Foot-and-mouth disease	Rhinovirus, Types A, O, C, SAT	Cattle, pigs, related species	Europe, Asia, Africa, South America	Contact exposure
Infectious hepatitis (human)	A-virus	Non-human primates	Worldwide	Contact exposure
Influenza and parainfluenza	Myxoviruses	Pigs, rodents, dogs and birds	Universal	Contact exposure. Animals rarely source for man

Lassa fever	Arenavirus	Rodents, others	Africa	Rodents, urine or contaminated dust, possibly man to man
Louping ill	Flavivirus/Group B	Sheep, less often cattle, sheepdogs. Rodents, deer, shrews, and red grouse may be carriers	Great Britain, Northern Ireland	Ticks (*Ixodes ricinus*)
Newcastle diseases	Paramyxovirus	Fowl	Universal	Occupational exposure (uncommon in man)
Pseudocowpox	Poxvirus	Cattle	Universal	Contact
Rabies	Lyssavirus	Carnivores and Chiroptera (bats)	Worldwide except Australia, New Zealand, Britain, Scandinavia, Japan, Taiwan (a number of smaller islands are also free)	Bites of diseased animals
Simian herpesvirus (B virus)	Herpesvirus	Rhesus monkeys	Widespread in Africa and Asia	Bites of monkeys, occupational exposure

was found to be gravy in a meat pie. Further minor outbreaks occurred in the UK in 1997. The bacteria responsible for these outbreaks (and others that have occurred in the UK and elsewhere in the world) is a toxin-producing strain of *E. coli* which causes severe abdominal cramps, diarrhoea, vomiting, haemorrhagic colitis and haemolytic uraemia leading to kidney and heart failure.

Escherichia coli can be found in all types of meat, as well as unpasteurised milk, eggs and some vegetables. It is transmitted to man through the consumption of raw or undercooked meat products and raw milk. Faecal contamination of water and other foods, as well as cross-contamination of food during preparation, can also lead to infection. Secondary transmission can occur via person-to-person contact by the oral–faecal route. It is certainly a fact that cattle are often 'dirtier' than in traditional systems of husbandry where there were copious amounts of bedding to absorb faecal and urinary excretions. Without this bedding, faeces adhere to the body and contaminate even the abbatoir environment.

There used to be two diseases of cattle which were a serious hazard to the human subject: tuberculosis and brucellosis. Both reached man largely via milk but have been adequately dealt with by the twin process of eliminating the disease from cattle and by pasteurising or sterilising the milk. Neither of these diseases now pose a hazard to man where the disease has been largely eliminated from the national herd, as in the UK and many other countries.

At the moment, however, these diseases are still present to a limited extent and their final elimination has not been achieved, hence cattle are still tested for tuberculosis at regular intervals. Before milk is infected the disease must be generalised and present in the udder and regular testing (or monitoring) will ensure milk or milk products are safe. It should be emphasised, however, that with proper cooking and hygiene in food preparation all risks are virtually eliminated in livestock products.

Parasitic infections

So far as parasitic infections are concerned, the dangers are few in this country. There are slight risks from ringworm in cattle and from a number of intestinal worms which can infect man either themselves or in their secondary forms. Under 'intensive' or housed conditions intestinal worms have almost been eliminated but it is likely there will be some increase in risk if the trend to outdoor husbandry systems continues and land is over-stocked and over-used. However, overall the risk is likely to remain minimal. It is pertinent to mention that it is unwise for absolute reliance to be placed on medication in the control of parasitic infections. It is better by far to consider medicines as adjuncts to good husbandry practices which could obviate their use altogether.

Viral infections

The list of viral infections of animals communicable to man is not vast but contains some which are very important. Bovine spongiform encephalopathy (BSE) is dealt with in detail later because of its enormous topical importance. Although it is classified here under viruses it is in fact thought to be due to an organism now known as a prion but which may also be termed a 'slow virus', an appropriate term in view of its very long incubation period.

Rabies is a virus infection of major importance but which rarely causes loss of human life nowadays. At present it is dealt with in the UK by a 6 month quarantine period for those animals which could bring it in and the national policy has enabled us to be free of all infection for some 30 years. In other countries, e.g. France, where rabies is present to a very limited extent in wildlife, susceptible domestic animals are dealt with by vaccination and the incidence in man is negligible. France has had one human rabies infection in 10 years.

In the UK a recently convened consideration of rabies by a House of Commons Select Committee made a strong and unanimous recommendation that the quarantine policy should be replaced by a compulsory vaccination policy. So far no action has been taken by the Government but it seems likely that before long a vaccination policy will be instituted to deal with the danger, now that we are an increasingly integrated part of the European Union.

The remainder of the viral infections listed in Table 4.3 tend to be either less serious or more probably associated with tropical or semi-tropical countries. Wherever the human subject goes the best procedure is to seek protection by vaccination, which can ensure freedom from infection for several years.

Arthropods

Fleas, mites, ticks and flies are capable of causing some disease in man but do not persist for very long as an infestation outside their natural hosts. They are certainly no more than a minor cause of trouble in themselves, but they can function in a zoonotic capacity as carriers of almost any disease. From a wealth of evidence, of which we have been aware for many years, diseases such as plague, tularaemia, haemorrhagic fevers, rickettsias and protozoal blood parasites can all be conveyed from animals to humans and between humans by arthropods but they tend to be more tropical or sub-tropical problems, rather than problems encountered in temperate climates.

Bovine spongiform encephalopathy (BSE) or 'mad cow disease'

There has been so much publicity and concern about this unique disease of cattle, which may be communicable to man, that a careful and detailed look at our present knowledge is more than justified.

Bovine spongiform encephalopathy (BSE) is an extremely serious disease of cattle, believed to have originated from infected meat and bonemeal in cattle feed concentrates, which was derived from a similar disease in sheep known as scrapie. The eradication of BSE is of vital importance to safeguard herds and hence the future supply of bovine meat and dairy products for human and animal food, together with important bovine by-products. In addition, it has been alleged that the consumption of infected bovine products may cause Creutzfeld-Jakob disease (CJD) in the human subject.

BSE is a fatal brain disease of cattle which has only come to light in recent years, having been first recognised in the UK in 1986. The incubation period for BSE is very long, commonly 3–5 years, but the range can be considerably wider, from 30 months to 8 years and possibly even longer.

From 1986 to the end of August 1996 there were 162 796 cases of BSE in cattle in the UK and the disease has also been confirmed in Ireland, Portugal, Switzerland, France and Germany, although the total elsewhere is said to be under 500 cases. The latter figure is surprisingly low considering that nearly 58 000 British breeding cattle were exported in the period 1985–1990, as were many thousands of tons of British meat and bonemeal.

The symptoms in cattle are as follows: the affected cattle appear to become extremely nervous, although there is no conventional madness. The cattle lost weight, have difficulty in walking and the milk yield declines markedly. However, confirmation of the disease is dependent on post-mortem examination of the brain tissue. Unfortunately, at the time of writing there is no certain test to detect the disease in live animals.

The risk to man

If there is a danger that BSE could be a risk to man, two situations must be considered: firstly, that the disease can be transmitted from cattle to man and, secondly, that parts of the diseased animals carrying the infective agent can enter the human food chain.

On the first issue, whilst it is certainly possible that it might occur, there is no direct scientific evidence to show that BSE can be transmitted from cattle to man. On the other hand, the emergence in the UK during the past 2 years of 17 anomalous cases of CJD caused by a new pathogen, previously unseen, led the Spongiform Encephalopathy Advisory Committee (SEAC) to the view that cases were most likely to have been caused by exposure of the affected people to infected brain or spinal cord before 1989, at which time they were banned from the food chain. This Committee also stated that if there is any risk to the human subject, it is extremely small and no greater for children, hospital patients, pregnant women or those people who are ill and lack the full power of their immunological systems. It is also fair to state that the possibility of this new type of CJD being contracted from cattle has no scientific backing and remains as conjecture.

The second issue is whether parts of a BSE-infected animal can enter the human food chain. The evidence at present is that whilst the BSE infective agent can be found in the brain, spinal cord and also the retina of affected cattle, extensive tests have failed to detect it in the muscle meat and milk of infected beasts. Mandatory measures have been taken, and strengthened, to prevent all those parts of the animal that might be infected from entering the food chain. The current enforcement of these regulations appears to be working efficiently, with heavy penalties being imposed by those who evade them, but very few people are doing so.

Therefore on the basis of the most up-to-date scientific work (a great deal more of which is still proceeding) and provided the above measures continue to be implemented, consumption of muscle meat, milk, gelatin and tallow from cattle in the UK should involve virtually no risk of causing CJD.

With regard to animal health, the measures taken have resulted in a dramatic reduction of BSE in cattle. It is expected there will be a virtual elimination of BSE within 3 years. Figure 4.3 shows the dramatic decline in cases and projects the likely position leading to the virtual elimination of the disease within 3 years.

The cause of BSE

Intensive research in recent years has confirmed that in neurodegenerative disorders such as BSE in cattle, scrapie in sheep and CJD in man, referred to collectively as transmissible spongiform encephalopathies (TSEs), the causative, infective agents are distorted, abnormal prions. A prion (PrP) is a small protein molecule found in the cell membrane, but which has no associated nucleii and so it is not classified as a living cell. The term 'prion' is a generic one and different species of animals have brain cell prion proteins of different compositions. For example, the amino-acid sequence of the human prion

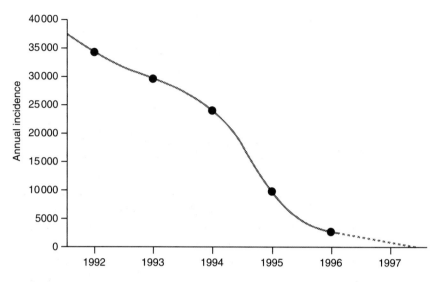

Fig. 4.3   Incidence and projection of BSE cases from peak in 1992.

differs at more than 30 positions from that of the cattle prion, whereas sheep
and cattle prions differ at only seven positions.

Let us consider what is believed to happen in the course of TSEs. The
molecule of a protein has a three-dimensional folded shape and an infective
prion is one with a distorted shape. This distorted prion is protease-resistant,
that is, it is not broken down into amino acids in the digestive system.

When one of these distorted prion molecules reaches the normal prions in
the brain the distorted molecule is able to act as a three-dimensional
'template' that makes a normal prion molecule of the same or a similar
composition to adopt a similarly distorted shape, which in turn acts as a
template to do the same to another normal prion molecule and so on. Since
only small quantities of brain cell prion are involved, the process can take a
very long time, hence the extraordinarily long incubation periods of TGEs.
It has been established from research that it is the *depletion* of the normal
brain prions rather than the deposition of distorted prions that is linked with
spongiosis, gliosis and neuronal death.

It is also pertinent to consider another TSE, namely scrapie of sheep.
Scrapie is a fatal brain disease of sheep and goats endemic in many countries
and it has been recorded in the UK for at least 200 years. It is naturally
transmitted between sheep and has an incubation period of between 2 and 5
years. There is no evidence that scrapie is transmitted to man either by
contact occupationally or by eating sheep meat or by-products. It is also
noteworthy that while scrapie is common in sheep, recorded CJD is very
rare in man and occurs in vegetarians as well as meat eaters. The incidence of

reported CJD is at a similar level throughout the world (around one million per year) regardless of the occurrence of BSE. The number of recorded cases of CJD in the UK fell from 55 in 1994 to 43 in 1995 and was even less in 1996.

Resistance to destruction of the prion

The various infective prions have a number of common characteristics. They are extremely resistant to heat and while some loss of infectivity occurs at temperatures above 100°C, temperatures greater than 120°C over long periods are needed to inactivate the finely divided material. Resistance to common sterilants and other chemical agents is very high, as is resistance to extremes of pH and to ultraviolet or ionising irradiation. The only chemical treatment so far found to be effective against all TSEs is sodium hypochlorite at 20 000 parts per million of available chlorine for 1 hour. It is believed that transmission of BSE has been by the oral route and BSE has been experimentally induced orally in several species. As pointed out previously, prions are not broken down in the intestines.

The origin of BSE in cattle

After the first cases of BSE appeared in 1986, when almost nothing was known about the disease, an epidemiological study of the first 200 cases indicated that the only factor in common had been commercial cattle feed concentrates which contained meat and bone meal (MBM) derived from sheep (and possibly cattle) presumed to have been infected with scrapie or BSE. This was said to have been coupled with a change in processing that eliminated a solvent extraction step and hence also eliminated a steam-stripping treatment that had been needed to remove solvent residues. This was a fine piece of epidemiological detective work and led to the banning of ruminant-based feed for ruminants.

Some experts have reservations about the sheep MBM hypothesis, particularly with regard to how the sheep scrapie prion changed, during passage through cattle, to the BSE prion. Some people offer the view that it has always existed, but occurred so rarely that when a cow had the 'staggers' nobody recognised it as anything but an inexplicable one-off local event. It has certainly been stated by several specialist veterinarians in the cattle world that they have seen a condition resembling BSE throughout their careers.

Likewise, subsequent research into inactivation of BSE infectivity indicates that the solvent extraction and steam-stripping procedures supposedly in operation until 1981 were not likely to have been effective in destroying infectivity. Furthermore the processing change was made by the largest renderers not in 1981, as was assumed, but in the early 1960s and not only in the UK.

It is possible that BSE developed in such large numbers as a result of a number of inciting factors coming into play in combination. There is currently a serious discussion among experts on the possible roles of exposure to organophosphorous compounds at sub-toxic levels, or of the possible role of hay mites as a vector.

Nevertheless, the prohibition of ruminant material from animal feed and the successive dramatic reductions in new cases over recent years (a 30% drop from 1993 to 1994 and more than a 42% drop from 1994 to 1995) seem to demonstrate that the animal feed was a key factor. The downward trend in the number of cases reported continued in 1996 when 7844 cases were confirmed compared to 14 298 in 1995, a 45% decrease.

Placental transmission has been proposed as a likely route for vertical transmission for scrapie in sheep (although the existence of vertical transmission of scrapie has been disputed) but placental transmission has not been demonstrated with BSE in cattle. Until recently, there has been no evidence of vertical transmission in cattle. A large-scale epidemiological study should have brought to light vertical transmission if it occurred, but it did not, which strongly suggests there is no significant occurrence.

Animal health controls

In the UK the principal measures for the control of BSE in cattle are:

(1) To slaughter animals clinically diagnosed on the farm. This has been enforced since 1988

(2) To prohibit the feeding of all material containing animal protein derived from ruminants to cattle and other ruminants since 1989; this has subsequently been extended since 1996 to its prohibition in food for all farm animals

(3) To incinerate all carcasses of cattle affected with BSE

The banning of ruminant material from ruminant feedstuffs from July 1988 obviously could not have any effect on animals already infected before that date, and due to the long incubation period it was inevitable that the disease would continue to develop for a few years after the ban. This was the main reason for the peak in numbers in 1992. However, of the total of 160 540 cases up to 31 May 1996, 27 177 cases were born after the ban (BAB), and were mostly born in the first 18 months after the ban, reducing to 119 born in 1992, one born in 1993 and none thereafter. The 'BAB effect' was due in part to farmers using up their stocks of cattle feed after July 1988 and in part to cross-contamination, in manufacture or on the farm, by the ruminant MBM feed used for other farm animals which was then still permitted. As a further step to ensure 100% compliance with the prohibition of MBM in feed, the UK Government is funding a scheme to recall and dispose of residual stocks of feed and feed ingredients from manufacturers and farms. Since 1 August 1996 the presence of mammalian MBM in any part of the feed chain, whether on farm, in transit or in feed mills, has been illegal with compliance audited by State Veterinary Service inspections. These actions are intended to ensure that the target of excluding BSE infectivity from cattle feed will be achieved as absolutely as possible.

The whole BSE, scrapie and CJD saga is difficult to comprehend and there are still many facts to be explained. A great deal of investigation is being undertaken in this country and abroad and it is likely that many new facts will emerge. Until the work is complete there will remain uncertainties and it is wise to keep an open mind to these.

The public is obviously seeking simple explanations and rapid solutions. Unfortunately, with a new and complex problem scientists have to search for answers, which are unlikely to be simple and which involve detailed research. The public also demands solutions to ensure absolute safety, which in fact is not possible in any aspect of life.

Nevertheless, we can say that from the present scientific evidence, and provided that the above-mentioned measures are fully implemented, muscle meat of British beef, milk and milk products, gelatin and tallow would appear to be without significant risk of causing CJD. These products are safe within the normal meaning of the term and BSE in cattle will eventually become extremely rare.

Conclusions: safety from stable to table

By almost any serious and unbiased analysis, livestock products in the UK are as safe as any in the world. Concentrated efforts continue to be made to ensure the freedom of livestock products from the primary infections. Auditing by independent, reliable authorities, together with government departments, means the position is monitored openly and honestly. Knowledge is increasing all the time on methods to keep food based on livestock products free of disease from 'stable to table' and whilst methods are by no means perfect and must constantly be under review and improved, great credit has to be given to the producers and the appropriate authorities in ensuring food safety. A huge number of monitored samples show that medicinal or other residues are not present at harmful levels, whilst freedom from contagious and infectious disease is generally equally well ensured. The use of illegal growth promoters or unsupervised or unauthorised medicines has rarely been found in the UK so it is with more than a little surprise that we find the media seizing on the slightest and flimsiest pretext to alarm the public over largely non-existent dangers in consuming livestock products. Whilst vegans and vegetarians make headway on the basis of false accusations and an irresponsible media, it should not be forgotten that humans are biologically omnivorous and a balanced diet is most easily achieved by a mix of vegetable and animal products. Vegetarian and vegan diets can have deficiencies, although these may be corrected by careful supplements.

Intensive animal production has both advantages and dangers but if one is aware of these they are no greater than with semi-intensive or extensive methods. Intensification enables good management and supervision. Animal care and veterinary supervision can be at its best indoors and so can the provision of feed and water and the protection of animals from predators. In many respects there are greater risks when the animals are outdoors.

On the debit side, animals kept intensively in large numbers (a large biological mass) present a risk that when disease does challenge them it may build up in virulence and, in the case of viruses, lead to a persistence that is very difficult to eliminate. It is for this reason that it is wise to limit the size of the unit and also to subdivide the enterprise so that appropriate depopulation and complete sanitation procedures can be regularly conducted. There are other great advantages in limiting the size of the enterprise: handling the livestock is easier and less disturbing; muck disposal is easier and indeed the muck may be used advantageously on the land surrounding the site and crops grown on the land can possibly help towards feeding the animals. In this way intensive animal husbandry is no longer a factory-like operation but becomes a part of agriculture which is environmentally friendly and an

Table 4.4 'From stable to table'. Ten measures to ensure livestock products are produced to ensure the consumer's safety.

(1) All accommodation and grazing periodically depopulated and cleaned.
(2) Appropriate hygiene applied to the buildings, equipment and site.
(3) After clearing and disinfection the procedures should be microbiologically monitored.
(4) The incoming livestock placed in the building should be monitored for the presence of any zoonotic pathogens.
(5) Vaccinations should be used wherever possible.
(6) No medicines or additives of any description should be used without veterinary or expert supervision and recording. Usage should be strictly limited.
(7) Any animal feed that could introduce infections should be checked and held until known to be safe.
(8) Drinking water should be tested and special attention paid to its freedom from pathogens. Continuous sanitising is advocated.
(9) All products should be monitored for safety before leaving the farm.
(10) Absolute security of the site from sources of infection must be ensured.

integrated part of the farm. By making use of the modern knowledge of disease control we can be assured of improving the health and well-being of animals and zoonoses may be no more than a memory of past times. Table 4.4 lists the ten major ways in which the zoonoses can be controlled.

Chapter 5

The Health of Cattle

Cattle have been as markedly affected by the trend towards intensive methods as most other forms of livestock and this has produced an inevitable crop of problems. At the same time traditional practices still persist alongside the more modern methods, so health problems arising from these remain. In this chapter the health problems are dealt with on a life-cycle basis, dealing firstly with those health problems affecting the calf and continuing with growing stock and concluding with the mature beast and those diseases that have no special age incidence.

The health of the calf

Of the 5–10% mortality that occurs in calves, nearly two-thirds takes place in the first month of life and a large proportion of this is due to what is usually referred to as calf scours. This is a rather vague term which covers a number of digestive and more generalised upsets. The main cause is ultimately the ubiquitous bacterium *Escherichia coli*, following earlier environment stress and usually viral challenges.

Colostrum and protection against diseases in the calf

It is always considered essential that a calf should have a good drink of colostrum (Table 5.1) shortly after birth. The importance of this can not be stressed too greatly as it provides so many benefits. The calf – or indeed any young animal – is virtually free of disease-causing organisms at birth. Colostrum contains the immunoglobulins and large quantities of Vitamin A (six times as much as in ordinary milk). Immunoglobulins are the proteins which contain the antibodies which protect the calf from disease organisms, whilst Vitamin A is the most important vitamin associated with the animal's resistance to infection.

The importance to the calf of having the colostrum is thus apparent but the speed of taking it in is of the essence for two reasons. First, the production of the best quality of colostrum is only a short-lived action and so

Table 5.1 Comparative levels of the main nutrients in colostrum as compared with ordinary cow's milk.

	Colostrum	Milk
Fat (g/kg)	36	35
Solids not fat (g/kg)	185	86
Protein	143	32.5
Immunoglobulins (g/kg)	55–68	0.9
Lactose (g/kg)	31	46
Iron (mg/kg)	2.0	0.1–0.7
Vitamin A (µg/kg)	42–48	8
Vitamin D (µg/kg)	23–45	15
Vitamin E (µg/kg)	100–150	20

is the absorption and assimilation by the calf of the elements needed to counteract infection. Second, colostrum must be given before the calf gets a bad challenge from disease-producing organisms, so that antibodies *precede* the infectious pathogens. The aim is for the colostrum to be taken within 1 hour of birth and the total consumption should be at least 2 kg.

Feeding systems for calves

There are a number of different systems for feeding calves. The choice is gradually increasing and each has advantages and drawbacks. The main systems are:

❑ Bucket feeding twice daily.
❑ Bucket feeding once daily – warm.
❑ Bucket feeding once daily – cold.
❑ Unrestricted warm milk.
❑ Unrestricted cold acidified milk.

Then there are a number of different powders that can be used to constitute the milk. Milk may be acidified to a pH of about 5.2, which preserves the material in an unrestricted cold milk feeding regime using teat feeders. There are low-fat milk replacers with 5–7% fat and up to 15–18% in the high-fat materials. Whilst all these methods show different results there is no clear evidence that there are any strong differences in their effect on health, but methods simulating the natural sucking of the calf from the teat are less likely to cause digestive upsets. Calves will react badly to sudden variations in their feeding regime so consistency is vital.

It should be stressed that calf scour (often called 'white scour') does not appear to be a simple infection with strains of *E. coli*. There is abundant evidence to indicate the effects of more than one viral agent, reoviruses and coronaviruses being some of those implicated. Under these circumstances the use of specific vaccines and sera may have a limited chance of providing good treatment or prevention, although sometimes this can be the case. More often the disease must be treated with antibiotics having a broad range of activity, such as the tetracyclines or synthetic penicillins, together with replacement therapy for the enormous fluid depletion that takes place. Replacement fluids include electrolytes, glucose, minerals and vitamins in easily assimilated liquid form. Treatment is not something for the amateur to undertake, especially when it is realised that mortality in affected calves can easily reach within striking distance of 100%.

Salmonellosis

The salmonella group of bacteria is a very large one with hundreds of different types, all potentially pathogenic to man and animals but some more than others and many specific only to certain hosts. However, only relatively few are very harmful, most being exotic types that come in via the feed and are quickly eliminated. Specific salmonella diseases are described in the consideration of each species in this book.

The two most important species in the condition in calves are *Salmonella typhimurium* and *Salmonella dublin*. The symptoms with either of these infections or indeed with other virulent salmonella can be largely similar. If a batch of calves is affected and there is close contact between them, then nearly all may be infected. A percentage may die so rapidly that no symptoms are seen; others scour profusely, with dysentery, pneumonia, arthritis, jaundice and nervous symptoms manifesting themselves in some cases. Extreme emaciation rapidly results if the calves live. Very recently a more virulent form of *S. typhimurium* has emerged with much enhanced pathogenicity.

Treatment will be required urgently if the calves are to be saved and is likely to include antibiotics, chemotherapeutics and fluid therapy, isolation and general nursing, especially warmth. Thorough disinfection of the quarters will be essential and preventive measures may include vaccination and possibly preventive medication. However, the use of the last measure is hazardous as it may generate drug resistance and encourage the establishment of a 'carrier' animal which can excrete salmonella organisms throughout its life.

Whilst salmonellosis is mainly a disease of young stock, adult cattle do become infected and may not show symptoms, becoming carriers of great potential danger to man and other livestock. Abortions may be caused by salmonella and salmonella can be a source of infection via milk. In the main the biggest problems from salmonellosis arise from farms where the calves are brought in from outside and infection can easily spread back to the adults if they are on the same premises. A recent worrying means of infecting calves and cows with salmonella is through the spread of slurry on the land. Salmonella can persist in slurry for months; if it is then spread over pasture which is about to be grazed it will be readily picked up by cattle, or indeed any animal that is on the ground.

In Great Britain salmonellosis is a notifiable infection and official measures can be taken to control the disease as appropriate. In the event of an outbreak in adult cattle, measures that may be taken include laboratory testing of the cattle to identify the carriers, treatment of animals with antibiotics such as enrofloxacin, amoxycillin or the tetracyclines and appropriate care of the milk to remove the risk of human infection.

Apart from the appropriate hygienic measures, the use of specific anti-sera and vaccines undoubtedly offer the most satisfactory methods of dealing with salmonella infections. At present there are a number of excellent biological products available for the most virulent types of salmonellosis and these should be resorted to, together with professional advice, wherever possible.

Calf diphtheria

The bacterium associated with foul-in-the-foot in cattle, known as *Fusobacterium necrophorum* is also capable of causing a serious disease in calves known as calf diphtheria. The infection attacks calves when very young, even as early as the third or fourth day of life, and causes inflammation within the mouth, leading to soreness, ulcers and ultimately necrosis. The calf becomes seriously ill, will not feed, salivates from the mouth and keeps on exhibiting swallowing movements. The course of the disease, if it is not checked at this stage, is progressive and the lesions will spread into the throat, necrosis will continue and there will be a characteristic foul smell. Without treatment most calves die.

The disease will respond very well to treatment. Sulphonamides are effective, as are a wide range of broad-spectrum antibiotics. It is a disease that is characteristic of bad hygiene so premises where this disease occurs should be thoroughly cleaned and thereafter management should be maintained at a higher standard.

Navel-ill or joint-ill

These two terms are jointly used to describe the diseases affecting calves where bacterial infection causes inflammation in the region of the navel, together with inflammation and lesions in the joints. The conditions that occur under this name are caused by a variety of bacterial organisms, common ones being *Corynebacterium pyogenes*, staphylococci, *E. coli, F. necrophorum, Pasteurella* and haemolytic streptococci. The disease usually occurs because the calves are managed under dirty conditions and are challenged by a serious burden of bacteria before the naval has healed.

Treatment may be undertaken successfully in the early stages of the disease with sulphonamides or broad-spectrum antibiotics; local application of dressings to the navel will help to prevent infection. It is important that any dressing so applied is not damaging to the delicate and fragile tissue of the area.

Some general points on the control of calf diseases

The moment a calf is born, or indeed even whilst it is being born, it will be subject to challenge from contagious or infectious disease. In any local community of animals on a farm a large number of organisms which are potentially pathogenic are present but normally these will not cause disease. Disease is only caused for a number of reasons, as follows:

(1) The calf may not have been born in the same environment as its dam was in during pregnancy so no immunity develops to local 'infections'
(2) The calf may not have received an adequate amount of the colostrum from its dam, the colostrum or first milk providing a major boost to the immunity of the calf to infections
(3) The premises may not have been cleaned and disinfected adequately so the calf will get an immediate and possibly overbearing contact with pathogenic microorganisms
(4) If young calves are put into housing that already contains a substantial number of older and infected or 'carrier' calves, the challenge imposed on the younger calves from the old stock can cause very serious losses

There are two main groups of diseases that affect calves – the enteric groups and the respiratory diseases. Management arrangements that avoid the stresses just listed will influence the likelihood of these two groups affecting the calves in a very real way (see Fig. 5.1 and also under *Calf tetany* later in this chapter). Table 5.2 sets out a 12-point plan for rearing healthier calves.

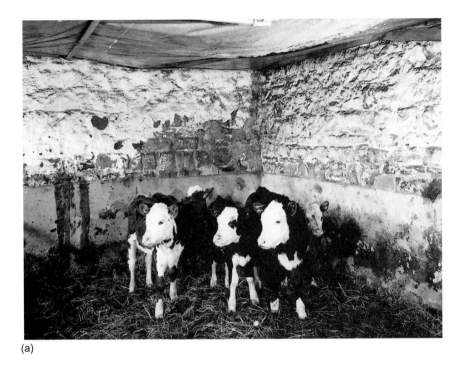

(a)

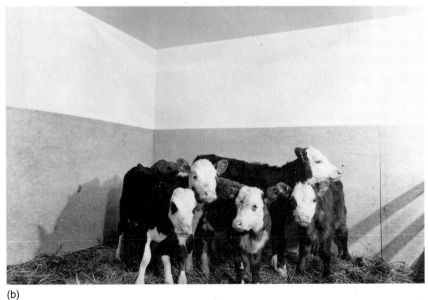

(b)

Fig. 5.1   Calf housing (a) before and (b) after improvement. The first picture shows a dirty surface, where cleanliness is only obtained with great difficulty, and sagging moisture-laden roof insulation. The second picture is with a new lining of fibre cement over polyurethane board insulation (Purlboard, ICI).

Table 5.2   A 12-point plan for rearing healthier calves.

(1) Place newborn calves in completely clean and disinfected pens
(2) Ensure they have colostrum immediately after birth and thereafter an adequate and balanced diet
(3) Isolate all calves moved on to the farm from outside for sufficient time to detect any disease – usually a few weeks
(4) Batch rear calves on the 'all-in, all-out' principle
(5) Small numbers should be kept in one common air space and with separation of dung between the sub-units
(6) Oppose movement and mixing of calves as far as economically possible
(7) Be generous with space allowances
(8) Provide free choice for the calves with a resting area warmer than the exercise and feeding area, as in 'kennel' housing
(9) Ventilation by natural methods is usually to be preferred if there is adequate air space. No draughts must be tolerated
(10) Provide enough insulation of the building surfaces to prevent condensation
(11) Separate different age groups wherever possible
(12) Remove sick calves and treat as speedily as possible

The health of growing cattle

Internal parasites

There are three major groups of diseases in cattle caused by parasitic worms. There is 'husk' or 'hoose,' which is due to worms which live in the lungs; parasitic gastroenteritis, which is caused by roundworms which live in the abomasum and/or intestine of cattle, and finally liver fluke disease, caused by flatworms or flukes, which live in the liver.

As a preliminary comment it needs to be emphasised that parasitic worms do not multiply within the body of the animal in which they live as adults. The adults produce millions of eggs which each individual worm can lay, but none reach maturity without first passing out of the animal with the faeces. They must then have a period of time outside the animal before they become infective, and this period varies from a few days to many weeks. Thus every worm in the animal has been picked up in the herbage while the animal was grazing; their mode of multiplication is entirely different from bacteria and viruses which multiply within the body. The significance of this knowledge is that it permits two means of attack, one within the body and one without. Removal of contact of animals with their own faeces is a vital factor. If the husbandry is good, with a clean environment and no over-crowding, the infestation may be so slight as to be unimportant. Mixed grazing is also useful since the parasitic worms are host-specific and infect only one species. It is also important to know that it is chiefly the young and growing stock that are vulnerable to infection. Adults should have a naturally produced immunity due to earlier contact with the parasites. Nevertheless, the adults can become reinfected if they become stressed by poor conditions or nutrition..

The worm eggs once voided can remain viable for some time. Some can remain in an infective form for up to or even more than a year. Resting of infected pasture is a very successful means of reducing the worm burden, and even a short rest will help.

Husk or hoose

When certain forms of parasitic worms infest the bronchi in the lungs this is often called verminous bronchitis. It is at first an infection of the bronchial tubes and leads to the cough known as 'husk' or 'hoose'. This condition is caused by the lungworm, *Dictyocaulus viviparus*. These white worms are threadlike and up to 75 mm long. They live in the bronchial tubes of the lungs and the females lay vast numbers of eggs (Fig. 5.2). After hatching, which soon takes place, they produce minute larvae which are carried in the mucus up the windpipe and to the mouth. They are then swallowed and pass out onto the pasture with the dung. These larvae have to develop on the ground before they are able to infect cattle, who take them in with the grazing. The development takes about 5 days in warm, moist weather and

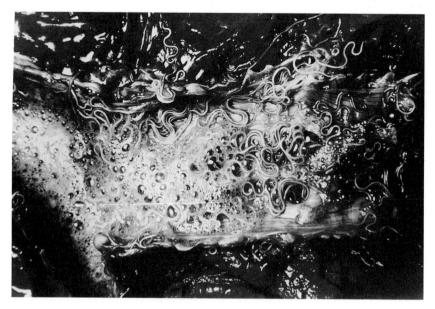

Fig. 5.2   Husk. A portion of a calf's lung showing adult lungworms 30 days after infection.

over a month when the weather is cold. Whilst developing in the dung the larvae go through a series of changes and moult their skins twice. The larvae have little resistance to drying and can die off rapidly under these circumstances. Figure 5.3 sets out the life cycle of the lungworm.

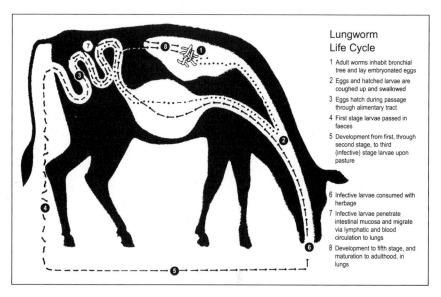

Fig. 5.3   The life cycle of the lungworm.

The season has a great effect on the infectivity of the larvae. In late spring, large concentrations of larvae may be found in the pasture but these generally die off quite rapidly. In summer, large concentrations are less likely to occur and equally unlikely to persist. Autumn conditions are ideal both for the creation of heavy infections on the pasture and for their survival. In winter it is very difficult for new infestations to be formed on the pasture but existing infestations do persist. Pasture can become infested quickly but does not remain so for long. The weight of infestation depends partly on the number of worms being carried out by the cattle that have grazed on it; the infestation in the herbage in turn determines how heavily calves grazing on it will become infested.

When the infective larvae are swallowed by grazing cattle they penetrate the intestinal wall and pass into the lymphatic system and by this route reach the blood stream and then pass to the lungs. Here they develop into the adult worms and begin to lay eggs after 3 weeks. These adults generally do not live long but small numbers may persist for a longer time and act as a continuing source of infection.

Cattle that have been exposed to lungworm infestation will in due course acquire a resistance; this resistance can develop quite rapidly but only as a result of sufficient infection. It thus follows that the number of lungworms which a susceptible calf picks up each day – depending on how heavily the herbage is infested – and the rate at which infection increases will determine whether the lungworm disease actually occurs.

If the level of pasture infestation rises at a moderate rate, the gradual and increasing resistance of the calf will enable it to reject the effect of the worms and no disease will actually occur. But if the pasture infestation rises rapidly, as it may do if the climatic conditions are favourable, disease may occur. The exposure of susceptible animals to a moderate uptake of larvae will produce symptoms of disease but will render the calves resistant so quickly that they are refractory to re-infestation. Exposing susceptible calves to a high rate of infestation will result in fatal disease. In all these cases the serious infection is acquired over a short space of time.

The situation in which a severe disease may appear can arise in a number of ways. The cattle may be insufficiently resistant either because they have not had sufficient exposure, as in the examples given above or they have lost their earlier resistance, having for some time been withheld from contact with infection. It is in these cases that adult cattle can be infected.

High pasture infestation may occur in a number of circumstances. In early spring most pastures will be either clean or at least only very slightly infested. Contamination of the pasture by older animals, which have carried over some worms in their lungs from the previous season, may produce more significant levels of infestation on the herbage and may even give rise to dangerous infestation if the season and pasture conditions are suitable. Low levels of herbage infestation may be increased when susceptible calves become infected on the pasture and in consequence increased numbers of larvae are passed on to it in their dung.

Symptoms

The disease may be recognised, or at least suspected, if there is an increase in the respiratory rate, coughing (especially when the animals are moved) and some loss in body condition. If cases become severe then the coughing becomes louder, the respirations shallow with clear pain and distress, and the animal stands uncomfortably with head and neck outstretched and the tongue protruding. There is anorexia and the beast may die within a few days. Post-mortem examination shows that parts of the lung have consolidated (liver-like in appearance) and the rest of the lungs seem water-logged and appear to be inflated with air and enlarged. The trachea and bronchial tubes are often filled with frothy mucus in which the worms can be seen. However, sometimes few adult worms are seen. Diagnosis may also be made in the absence of post mortems, since examination of the dung in the laboratory will show the presence of the larvae of the worms.

Control

The worms in the lung tend to be established in bronchial mucus or in the exudate caused by their presence. It is thus rather difficult for a medicine to reach the worms because of the protection this mucus affords. There are, however, a number of useful drugs for lungworms, such as doramectin, ivermectin, levamisole and oxfendazole. However, it should be emphasised that removal of the worms by medicines does not necessarily cure the condition since it may take a long time and good nursing to effect recovery. The best procedure is really to remove the animals from the pasture altogether and house the cattle in warm, dry, well-ventilated buildings where they can be well fed.

Prevention

Obviously the important lesson to be learned from an outbreak is how to prevent the condition in the future. The control depends on establishing and maintaining a state of immunity in the animals and yet avoiding outbreaks of disease. It is, of course, difficult to get such a controlled exposure without causing a disease, although modest rates of stocking are always likely to be of help. It is wise to keep animals grazing for their first year off pasture which has had animals on it recently. Strict systems of rotational grazing can always be of help since they will prevent heavy build-ups of disease. The calves should be moved twice a week on to ground which has not had calves on it for about 4 months, but even a shorter time would be of help in reducing infection. The vaccine which is available is also of great help in preventing the disease. This consists of infective-stage larvae which have been subjected to irradiation, a procedure that prevents the larvae from migrating into the lungs to produce disease but which does induce some immunological response. Thus it is an *adjunct* to good management but not a substitute.

Liver fluke disease

Liver fluke disease tends to go quite undetected or unsuspected until the animals start dying. It is admittedly more a disease of sheep than cattle but there is good evidence that liver fluke disease causes a very serious effect on growth and productivity. It can affect beasts outside at all ages and control should be taken very seriously. The liver fluke is a flat worm about the size and shape of a privet leaf. The worm lives and feeds on the liver of cattle. The flukes lay many thousands of eggs and they pass on to the pasture in the dung. The eggs hatch and produce a very small swimming creature but this, however, exists for no more than a day. If it is going to survive it must enter a particular type of snail and this snail must therefore be present for the disease to go on regenerating. The parasite grows in the liver of the snail and produces many young liver flukes. These look like the flukes which cause disease in the older stock, except that they are much smaller. These young flukes leave the snail when the snail is in water and surround themselves with a protective covering. They remain as cysts on the herbage but are inactive for long periods – up to months on occasion – until eaten by the grazing animal. When eaten the protective coat disappears and the fluke emerges and makes its way to the liver. During the next 2–3 months the fluke grows to maturity and then lays eggs (Fig. 5.4)

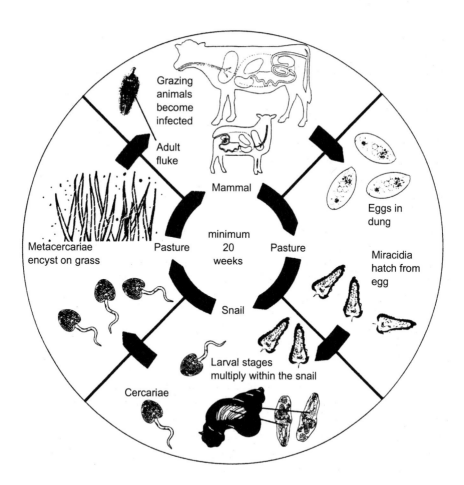

Fig. 5.4   The life cycle of the liver fluke parasite.

Symptoms

There are two forms which are clinically differentiated. The acute disease occurs when the grazing animal picks up many flukes in a short time. These damage the liver seriously and this can lead to sudden death in the apparently healthy animal. A post mortem may show a liver which is actually ruptured and the surface pitted with white tracks. The chronic form is quite different and much more serious and common. It is due to the presence of flukes in the liver over a period of several months and affected animals waste during this time. If nothing is done to allay this state of affairs, the cattle will die. Post mortems show their livers to have a 'pipey' look due to the thickening of the bile ducts and they may contain hard and stony deposits.

Such symptoms can occur only if cattle have been grazing on ground moist enough to support the snail; this will be badly drained ground. The disease tends to occur only in those years when the climatic conditions favour the secondary hosts.

Control

Certain drugs now exist for treatment, namely oxyclozanide, nitroxynil, albendazole and rafoxanide. Professional advice should generally be sought before use of these drugs in view of possible side-effects, contra-indications and withdrawal periods of milk for human consumption.

The disease can be effectively prevented by controlling the secondary hosts – the snails. Infestation in flukey areas is worse in the months of October to December and hence fluke-free pastures should be grazed during this period wherever possible. Badly drained areas should be properly drained. The snails may also be dealt with by treating the pasture with either copper sulphate at 30 kg/hectare or sodium pentachlorphenate at 10 kg/hectare. As these are dangerous materials they should be applied with care. A safer material is N-tritylmorpholine.

Parasitic gastroenteritis

This is a disease, or infestation, caused by the presence of a group of small roundworms in the abomasum or fourth stomach or the anterior part of the small intestine. Twenty-six species of roundworms have been identified in the alimentary tract of cattle in Great Britain. The most important species are *Ostertagia ostertagi, C. punctata, Trichostrongylus vitrinus* and *T. colubriformis* in the small intestine and *Oesophagostomum radiatum* in the large intestine. There is every evidence that they are equally a problem in other countries. They cause considerable economic loss from both poor productivity and overt disease, chiefly in young animals but not excluding older ones. Some are large enough to be seen in the stomach contents with the naked eye, whilst others are almost impossible to recognise in this way.

The life cycle of the worm is 'direct'; there being no intermediate hosts. Eggs are laid by the adult worms passing out with the dung on to the pasture where they can hatch within about 24 hours, producing minute larvae which feed on bacteria in the faeces. Within the next few days they moult twice and only then are they capable of infesting stock which ingest them in the herbage. In order to make the ingestion more certain they leave the dung and pass on to the grass, climbing upwards so that they will be readily consumed by the animals. All this can take less than 4 days in warm, damp weather, but may take weeks in cool conditions. The infective larvae can resist adverse weather quite well though they 'like' cold, dampish conditions but perish fairly readily when the weather is hot and dry. Most larvae will live for only 6-8 weeks but a few can survive for up to a year.

A limited number of worms do little or no harm to the beasts but a heavy infestation can be very damaging or even lethal. Thus infestation is assisted by overcrowding, moist, warm conditions and long grass in which moisture more readily persists. Adult cattle are generally resistant but this is only because they have normally been exposed to the worms early in life and have acquired an immunity.

Symptoms of parasitic gastroenteritis

These are nearly always indefinite and the usual signs are a progressive loss of condition, possibly leading to emaciation and death. There is usually a severe scour but the animals continue to eat voraciously. The disease should be suspected from these signs when a substantial number in a herd are showing them. However, one should be aware of the fact that some animals will not scour and signs can be so indefinite as to go undetected. In every case it is wise to have positive indentification by examining the faeces to determine the degree of infection.

Control

The first course of action is to consider medication, and there are a wide variety of materials that can be given: doramectin, ivermectin, benzimiadoles and levamisole. These drugs can be administered by injection or orally in several cases and a full course, as advised in the specific literature for the drug, should be given.

Preventive measures should consist of the following:

❑ Overcrowding of the young stock should be avoided
❑ Grass should be kept short as larval worms tend to perish in such grass
❑ Only adult stock should be put on badly infested land

❏ Periodic treatment should be given to animals after laboratory examination of faeces has established the degree of infection.

Parasitic gastroenteritis in adult cattle

It has long been assumed that adult cattle are not affected to any extent with parasitic roundworms as they have developed an immunity during their rearing period. In recent years, however, evidence has accumulated to show that this is not necessarily so.

The symptoms of infestation with these parasites tend to be insidious and may be so slight as to go undetected. Trials have shown that after treatment of cows with anthelmintics milk yield may increase considerably.

The best methods of control integrate grassland management and chemotherapy. At present, herbage availability regulates grazing systems rather than helminthological considerations. In fact, because they have a low, faecal egg output, adult cattle are often used to reduce the level of pasture contamination prior to its being used by younger stock, but this is a thoroughly dangerous arrangement.

Skin conditions and external parasites

Ringworm

This is an extremely common skin disease of cattle which tends to be a problem in winter when the animals are housed. It is caused by fungi belonging to the genus *Triochophyton*, two species of which occur in cattle in this country and also attack horses, pigs, dogs and man. *Trichophyton verrucosum* is the most common one and is responsible for most cases of ringworm in cattle, farmers, stock-keepers and their families, whilst *T. mentagrophytes* is very rare in cattle and occurs mostly in cats and dogs.

The fungi that cause ringworm are capable of surviving for very long periods in the farmyard, certainly for over a year and probably much longer. The spores that are picked up by the animals find their way into cracks on the skin and germinate to produce fine filaments which flourish in the surface of skin and hair. These fungal threads grow downwards inside the hair, keeping pace with its growth from the hair bulb and weakening it so that it snaps off at the surface of the skin producing the characteristic bald areas. The skin reacts to the infection by inflammation followed by the formation of a grey to yellow–white crust. The lesions of ringworm are most often seen on the head and neck, especially in calves, but in adults patches can occur on the flanks, back and rump, wherever rubbing takes place. Animals that are run-down are especially likely to suffer a severe infestation but ringworm itself does not seem to have a very harmful effect on animals.

Also, recovery usually happens spontaneously, often taking place after winter-housed animals are turned out to grass. Cattle that have recovered from ringworm are immune to further infection.

Control of ringworm

Whilst ringworm will disappear spontaneously in the course of time, it is never advisable to ignore treatment since the disease has a further debilitating effect on animals that may already be in low condition. Treatment may be done by dressing the affected areas with imidazoles preparations, for example 5% thiabendazole, handling with care, wearing rubber gloves and overalls. However, an antibiotic known as griseofulvin is now available for dosing animals with this condition.

The medicine is absorbed into the tissues of the body and is incorporated into newly formed skin and hair so that the growth of the fungus in these tissues is prevented. The bald patches rapidly improve and new hair appears within 2–3 weeks of commencing treatment. Griseofulvin must be given every day for some 3 weeks to produce a cure. This is a considerable expense so that in general only the most valuable stock are dealt with in this way. A much more important and economic approach is to practise good hygienic measures by efficient cleansing and disinfection of the buildings and all objects that could harbour the fungal spores. In the same way, consideration should be given to anything capable of transmitting infection, such as grooming tools. It is worth noting that most farmers do not bother to deal with this disease at all, accepting it as a normal happening in young housed cattle, but this ignores the debilitating effect of the infection which in trials has been shown to be harmful.

Mange

Certain forms of mites infect cattle: *Sarcoptes scabei, Chorioptes bovis, Psoroptes communis* and *Demodex bovis*. All are extremely contagious conditions (sometimes called scabies). The result of the disease is to produce very patchy coats and areas of bare skin with an extreme amount of irritation.

The nature of the disease is as follows. The mites spend their whole lifetime on the animals and only survive a few weeks off them. The symptoms are always at their worst during the final winter months. Diagnosis is made by microscopic examination of skin scrapings. The mites are just visible to the naked eye.

The most severe form of mange is caused by sarcoptes. This mange parasite is a white, tortoise-shaped mite with eight stumpy legs (Fig. 5.5). It burrows deeply into the outer layers of the skin, causing intense irritation, while the mites form the tunnels in which the females lay their eggs. The larvae which hatch from the eggs resemble the adult but are smaller and have

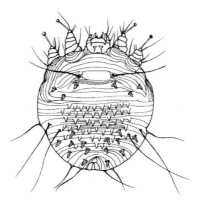

Fig. 5.5   Dorsal view of *Sarcoptes scabei* mite (× 100) which causes mange in cattle.

only six legs. These larvae moult and develop into eight-legged nymphs. Another moult takes place and within about 15 days from the laying of the egg a new generation of adults is produced. This species of mite spends nearly all its life under the skin of the animal so that it is difficult for insecticides to get to it.

The mites multiply very rapidly and spread out from the original area of infection. The most badly affected parts are often the groin and belly, whence it spreads to the head, neck and limbs. If the disease is allowed to spread it may affect all parts of the body. The burrowing of the mites and the bacterial invasion which accompanies it have a very serious debilitating effect. This type of mange also affects other animals and man, in the latter case the disease is called 'Dairyman's itch'.

Other types of mange are probably more widespread. Mange due to *Chorioptic scabei* is a very widespread condition but this mite does not burrow under the skin; it spends its whole existence among the scabs it produces on the surface of the skin. It therefore tends to be much less irritating and harmful. Psoroptic mange is similar, being less severe than the sarcoptic form.

Control
Control is rather difficult and requires professional veterinary advice. Any incidence should first be identified and once this has been done measures can be advised to eradicate the disease from the herd. Amitraz and ivermectin, certain organo-phosphorous compounds and synthetic pyrethroids can be applied. All animals should be treated and in order to eradicate the condition it will be necessary to re-treat two or three times at 10-day intervals. It is also necessary to keep the cattle away from those parts of the building that could harbour the mites and/or disinfect these areas as effectively as possible to prevent re-infestation.

Blackquarter (blackleg)

The disease of blackquarter is similar to so-called blackleg of sheep. It is caused by a bacterium called *Clostridium chauvoei* the spores of which are common inhabitants of the soil in areas where sheep and cattle have long been grazed. It is equally common on permanent pasture as on uncultivated, low-lying damp soils. In general, drainage and cultivation will reduce or destroy the spores.

The disease occurs because the organism is able to multiply in the muscles of the leg. The symptoms are stiffness and lameness with swellings appearing in areas such as the loin, buttocks or shoulder. The swellings are hot and painful at first but later the swellings become cold and painless. The skin over the affected muscles will become hard and stiff and if pressure is applied there is a papery effect – a dry, crackling noise due to the stiffness of the skin and movement of the gas underneath. In fatal cases the condition of the animal rapidly deteriorates and it will die quite quickly. So far as one can tell there is possibly initially some bruise or injury in the muscle and it is in this area that the clostridia can multiply in the absence of oxygen, then they produce the toxins which have the serious destructive effect on tissues.

Animals affected with the disease can be treated successfully with antibiotics only if the disease is recognised very early on. Preparations based on penicillin are suitable. Prevention can be affected by using a vaccine but the best measures of prevention rely on good pasture management, avoiding areas of known susceptibility and draining or cultivating those that must be used.

Coccidiosis in cattle

Coccidiosis is a form of dysentery that primarily affects young stock in the summer and autumn months. It is caused by a microscopic unicellular parasitic organism known as a coccidium. The coccidial parasite forms spores that can live outside the animal for many months. Adults are frequently carriers of the coccidial parasites but show no symptoms, yet spread the disease to younger animals. There are a large number of different species of coccidia, at least four types infecting cattle, and each causing rather different symptoms.

The adult coccidia produce masses of microscopic spores which are passed out in the dung and under favourable warm and wet conditions mature in a couple of days and can then infect other animals. The oocysts are very resistant to destruction and can often remain infective for a year, but if swallowed by a susceptible animal they hatch and the active forms of the coccidia are liberated. These coccidia penetrate the cells lining the intestine where they mature and multiply. Thus, they affect a considerable amount of the intestinal wall and break down areas of the mucosa, causing diarrhoea and bleeding, which is the characteristic symptom at this time. After a period of multiplication many oocysts are formed and are passed out with the faeces to infect the pasture or the bedding wherever the animals are housed.

Animals acquire a resistance to coccidiosis by receiving a light infestation early in life and developing an immunity. However, if the intake of oocysts is sudden and too great at any one time before a resistance has been produced, disease will occur. This is most liable to happen where animals are densely stocked and the weather conditions are warm and wet. Dirty walls of pens or boxes, as well as the floor, are common sources of infection. In addition to moisture and warmth, the oocysts also require air for their development in the dung so small amounts of faeces on the wall of the pen are very dangerous because of the aeration they receive. Oocysts often ripen particularly well on the coats of cattle and can be readily licked off by calves.

Symptoms are bad diarrhoea with evidence of bleeding and strings of mucus in the dung. In severe cases the animal also strains with its back in a characteristically arched position. The affected animal usually develops a strong thirst and rapidly loses condition and becomes weak; death can all too often follow.

The disease is controlled in a number of ways. Affected animals should be treated with a suitable medicine, such as sulpha compounds or amprolium, plus plenty of really good nursing, especially fluids. It may also be necessary to carefully consider the hygienic standards of management, but it should not be the intention of management to try to totally prevent any access of oocysts; this would be impossible and potentially dangerous as the animals would have no resistance at all and would rapidly succumb when challenged with oocysts.

Overstocking must be avoided; good bedding and cleanliness are important, and animals should be kept in good thriving conditions so that they can readily resist any infection that occurs.

Bovine virus diarrhoea (mucosal disease)

Bovine virus diarrhoea (BVD) or mucosal disease (MD) is an infectious disease of cattle caused by a virus. It was first recognised in the USA but in recent times it has occurred in virtually all parts of the world. Originally the diseases BVD and MD were distinguished between but it is now clear that they are caused by the same virus so the best term is probably BVD–MD complex. The evidence is that this is an increasingly pathogenic condition and professional advice is required to deal with it. This may well involve blood testing the herd and removing those persistently excreting the virus.

Symptoms

The disease causes ulceration of the mouth and lips accompanied by foul-smelling diarrhoea. There is often lameness and extreme scurfiness of the skin. By far the majority of cases occur in cattle between 4 and 18 months of age. Most cases can recover spontaneously but exceptionally if many young animals are affected the death rate can be high.

Treatment and control

There is no specific treatment but supportive therapy in the form of intestinal astringents and electrolytes can be of value. Vaccines are obtainable in some countries but are not evidently of very much use.

Infectious bovine rhinotracheitis (IBR)

This is an acute respiratory disease of cattle caused by a virus and is spread by contact or by the air-borne route. It is a very contagious disease and can spread through a herd within 7–10 days.

Symptoms

The symptoms are of severe inflammation of the eyes and the upper respiratory tract. The disease can also cause a substantial fall in milk yield, abortion and infertility. There may be a fever, loss of appetite and drooling of the saliva; sometimes there is a pronounced cough.

Control

IBR should always be looked upon as a serious condition; it can be treated with broad-spectrum antibiotics to help reduce pyrexia or the effect of secondary invaders. A vaccine is available to protect the herd.

Respiratory diseases in cattle

The dangers of disease inherent in intensive systems of housing cattle, which puts large numbers of beasts of all ages in very concentrated conditions, have already been alluded to in Chapter 1. The number of pathogenic organisms that can infect the respiratory system of cattle is enormous: there are some 20 bacteria, six fungi, and four parasites that *commonly* infect them, not to mention the underlying primary damage that may be wrought by viruses. The wide involvement of so many agents has made the production of satisfactory vaccines most difficult and the use of drugs complicated and expensive. Thus the prime responsibility for dealing with such conditions rests with achieving the correct environment.

The general principles have already been given in Chapter 1. Specific advice for cattle may be summarised as follows:

(1) Depopulate between batches and institute a rigid disinfection programme
(2) Reduce numbers in one environment to a minimum
(3) Keep different ages and sizes of animals separate
(4) Ensure copious ventilation without draught as cattle are hardy animals and do not require cosseting

Good ventilation is particularly important and the diagrams in Fig. 5.6 illustrate the ways this is achieved using various forms of housing. Figures 5.7–5.9 show examples of well-ventilated cubicle houses.

Diagram A in Fig. 5.6 shows the type of ventilation suitable for a totally enclosed cattle building with chimney trunk ventilator on the roof and hopper air inlets. Diagram B shows the details of the trunk ventilator and regulating flap, which are important. Diagram C is a ventilating open ridge for all types of cattle yard, a vital component for proper air flow, whilst Diagram D is a detailed drawing of the hopper inlet. With Monopitch buildings the best arrangement is a hopper inlet at the rear and a full-width ventilating flap at the front (Diagram E). The yard should face south.

With cattle yards it is difficult to have too much ventilation but it must be without causing draughts and two excellent ways of assisting this are to use spaced boarding (Diagram G) and the breathing roof (Diagram F), the latter being an arrangement whereby the roof sheets are placed upside down, with a 15 mm gap between them, thus giving ventilation all over the area of the yard. It is a very good system for wide yards with a shallow pitch on the roof. Table 5.3 provides dimensions essential for the provision of a sufficient outlet area for cattle and includes other farm livestock for reference. Table 5.4 likewise gives the ventilation rates to be used wherever mechanical arrangements are used.

A check list of essentials in countering respiratory disease outbreaks is given in Table 5.5

Wooden tongue and lumpy jaw

These are two distinct diseases which have rather similar symptoms and are

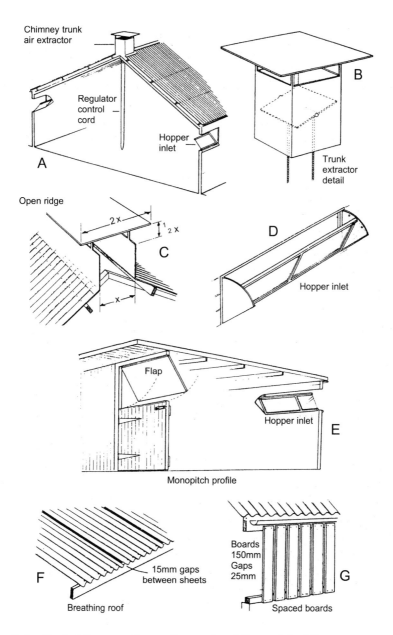

Fig. 5.6 Typical features of naturally ventilated livestock buildings.

caused by unrelated organisms. They both run a slow course and are characterised by a steady enlargement of the tongue and swellings in various parts of the animal, but especially on the head and neck. Their presence may generally interfere with the normal functions of the animal – they can also ulcerate or burst an abscess, discharging into or outside the body. Untreated

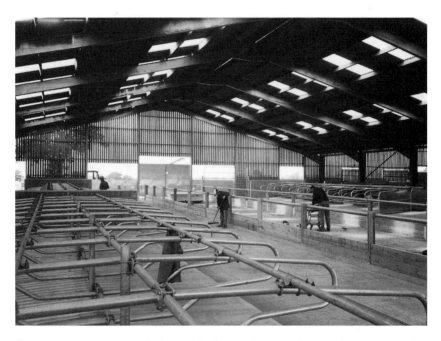

Fig. 5.7   Interior view of a large cubicle cow house. The ventilation is provided by generous amounts of boarding, which is usually 150 mm wide with gaps up to 20 mm. Note the spaced boarding (also called 'Yorkshire boarding') at the gable ends and sides of the yard.

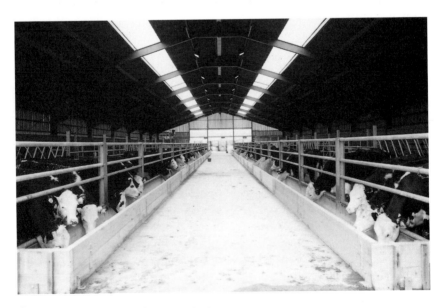

Fig. 5.8   A strawed cattle yard which is well ventilated and with a wide central passage allowing easy feeding into the troughs.

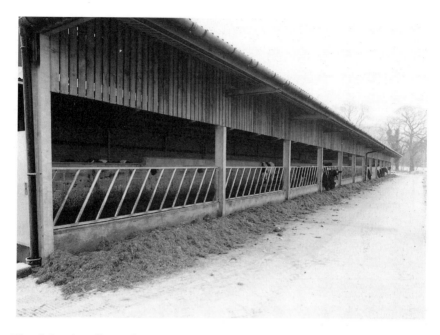

Fig. 5.9 A well ventilated cattle building with a good overhang on the roof to prevent excessive rain or snow entering and spaced boarding over the upper half to provide good ventilation.

they cause a steady wasting of the animal so that it becomes unproductive and will eventually die.

The cause of the two diseases are quite different. Actinomycosis is caused by a ray fungus known as *Actinomycetes bovis*, whereas actinobacillosis is caused by a bacterium *Actinobacillus ligneresi*. The main difference between the two diseases is that actinobacillosis tends to affect the soft tissues, such as the tongue, and actinomycosis usually causes diseases of the bones, especially those of the jaw.

Table 5.3 Minimum area for the outlet of stale air in farm buildings.

Type of building	Minimum outlet area m^2 per animal
Cows	0.09
Farrowing pigs	0.01
Fattening pigs	0.008
Calves	0.006
Laying birds	0.003
Broiler poultry	0.0015

Table 5.4   Ventilation rates for varying conditions in temperate climates for farm livestock.

Animal	Ventilation rate (m³/hour per kg body weight)	
	Maximum summer rate	Minimum winter rate
Adult cattle	0.75–1.4	0.19
Young calf	0.94–1.9	0.38
Sow and litter	0.94–1.9	0.38
Fattening pig	0.94–1.9	0.38
Broiler chicken	2.8–4.7	0.75
Laying poultry	5.6–9.4	1.50

Table 5.5   A check list of essentials in countering respiratory disease outbreaks in cattle.

Expert attention required for correct therapy
Improve ventilation – usually needed are more air flow and less draught
Check stocking density – are the cattle overcrowded?
Is more bedding required?
Separate and, if possible, isolate those cattle that are badly affected
Provide warmth for the very sick
Attempt separation of different ages
Reduce movement of animals to a minimum
Consider insulation and other essentials of construction relevant to the building
Can serum, vaccine or medicines be used to protect the unaffected animals?

Symptoms

These depend on the organs affected and the seriousness of the disease depends largely on the importance of the affected part. Nodules of various sizes, usually hard to the touch, may form in the skin of the head and neck; at other times the skin becomes broken and the nodules are soft, yellow in colour and with a covering of crust.

The tongue is most commonly affected and becomes hard and rather rigid, thus the name 'wooden tongue'. There is a constant dribbling of saliva and food tends to be rejected. The tongue is also very sensitive and painful. The disease will also affect the glands of the neck and a swelling appears between the angles of the jaw. If this swelling is allowed to continue it will affect breathing and swallowing also becomes difficult. The lesions may burst and release a characteristic yellow and granular pus. In addition the bones of the jaw are often affected as a result of the fungus growing into the bone from the soft parts of the mouth, possibly through the sockets of the teeth.

Pus forms within the bone and these diseased areas can eventually break through the skin to form an unpleasant discharging fistula.

These are, however, the external signs of the diseases. They may also affect the internal organs and will then cause a progressive wasting.

Control and treatment

Other than in advanced cases, treatment can be very successful. If it does seem to have got a firm hold on the animal which is fast losing condition, it is probably best to cull it. Actinobacillus responds quite well to iodides, streptomycin and sulphonamides and actinomycosis will be suitably treated with broad-spectrum antibiotics. Very careful veterinary supervision will be needed if the measures chosen are to be satisfactory.

Prevention of the disease is best achieved by responding quickly to any wounds on the face of cattle and elsewhere by dressing with an appropriate antibacterial material. There is no preventive vaccine available.

Redwater

Redwater, also called bovine piroplasmosis or babesiosis, is a curious condition caused by the presence in the blood of minute parasites called piroplasms. These parasites live inside the red blood corpuscles where they can be seen in the early stages of the disease. It is a condition that tends to be found in certain well-defined areas; in the British Isles, for example, it occurs mostly in Wales and south-west England and small areas of East Anglia.

Piroplasmosis is a much more serious disease in tropical countries than in the UK where only one species of the parasite is present. This is *Babesia divergens* and its presence is associated with rough scrubland or on heathland or woodlands where ticks are present. The condition is transmitted from animal to animal by the tick *Ixodes ricinus*, which acts as a carrier. The tick is infected by sucking the blood of an infected animal. Once the tick is engorged with blood it falls off and lies in the herbage. Later the tick may attach itself to other cattle and when it sucks from these it introduces the parasites into their blood. The ticks may be seen on the animals, often in considerable numbers. During the life cycle of the tick it feeds on three separate animals, first as a larva, then as a nymph and finally as an adult. At each stage it feeds on blood and when full falls to the ground in order to digest its meal and grow. It is probable that infection is transmitted at each stage. Infected adult ticks pass on infection through to the new generation via the egg. Thus an infection can remain within a tick population for a long while, even in the absence of cattle.

Symptoms

The two worst periods for redwater disease are from March to June and October to November. The main effects of the disease are to cause loss of condition and a very considerable loss of milk yield. The disease is characterised by the presence of the dark blood pigment in the urine of the affected animals, but this symptom is not invariably present. Sometimes there is very little discoloration or in others the urine may turn black. There is always an increase in urine.

Animals affected also show a high fever and diarrhoea and later constipation. The animal also often becomes jaundiced; the mucous membranes becoming yellow. The heartbeat becomes very loud and there are tremors of the muscles of the shoulder and legs. Temperament also often changes for the worse. In the later stages of the disease the animal becomes dull and listless, anaemic, the urine darker and death may take place.

Many of the symptoms are induced by the destruction of the red blood corpuscles by the parasites and the release of the red colouring matter. Much of this escapes into the urine via the kidneys, causing the typical 'redwater' and damaging the kidneys. The jaundice and the extra exertion of the heart are also associated with this same factor. It should be noted that young cattle are less susceptible than adults which have not previously been infected. If contracted early in life the disease is only mild and the animal is then immune against further infection. This indicates one of the great dangers; if adult cattle from a tick-free area are introduced into a redwater area, some of these may contract the infection and die quite rapidly without treatment.

Control

Treatment of infected animals will be two-fold. First, the animal will require injection with one of a number of chemotherapeutic agents that are lethal to the parasite, such as Piroparv. It is important that these are given to the animal early in the course of the infection. Second, careful nursing is perhaps even more important: feed well, house comfortably, do not drive or excite for fear of heart failure and keep the animal warm.

The recovered animal usually retains the infection and this is a carrier of the disease. This small degree of infection thereby protects the animal by ensuring that the body's immunological system is always 'alert'. Indeed, in redwater areas the usual thing to happen is for a young animal to contract the disease mildly and thus acquire protection. This procedure is often good but there are certain inherent dangers in relying on this immunity. The resistance of these animals may be broken down by a sudden change of weather or any other circumstance that can lower the general condition of the animal. It is difficult to know which animals are protected and which remain fully susceptible. Thus if animals are newly introduced into a redwater area herd from outside then they must be very carefully watched for signs of redwater for several weeks.

Prevention

The disease could be eradicated if ticks were eliminated. The tick is extremely resistant to most measures of control. In addition it can feed off several species of animal and is not dependent on cattle alone. Sometimes sheep are put on pasture as 'tick collectors'. Placing them alone on the pasture at the worst tick seasons of the year and then adopting a heavy dipping programme reduces numbers considerably. The only effective way of eliminating ticks is to clear the rough ground by cultivation and normal crop rotation.

Wherever this procedure is adopted and a part of the farm is freed from ticks, the importance of exposing young animals to tick infestation must be considered, otherwise they will be highly susceptible to a first infection as adults. Great care must be taken not to put them on to tick-infested ground for the first time in adulthood.

Diseases of mature cattle

Bovine spongiform encephalopathy (BSE) or mad cow disease

This is a recently recognised progressive neurological disorder affecting adult cattle, mainly dairy cattle, in mainland Britain, Orkney, the Channel Islands, Northern Ireland, Saudi Arabia, France and Switzerland. Sporadic cases have also occurred in other countries.

Symptoms

BSE is characterised clinically by behavioural changes and pathologically by vacuolation of the neuropils and some nuclei of the brain stem. The pathological changes resemble those of certain other neurological disorders collectively known as the transmissible spongiform encaphalopathies and classified among the 'slow virus' diseases. It affects cattle of 3–6 years of age. The initial signs are subtle and include persistent grinding of the teeth and repetitive, agitated, purposeless movements of the head and limbs. Affected animals become increasingly apprehensive and may become aggressive when approached. A sudden noise may result in the animal collapsing into a tetanic spasm. The course of the disease varies between 2 weeks and several months. A presumptive diagnosis can be made on the clinical signs, although in the early stages of the disease it may be confused with acetonaemia, hypomagnesaemia or listerial encephalitis. Confirmation of diagnosis can be made following a neuropathological examination.

Cause

The agent causing BSE is not firmly established. It appears to be an infective particle, sometimes suggested to be a novel kind of infectious protein or 'prion', which is highly resistant to physical or chemical disinfection, such as boiling, exposure to formalin or ultraviolet radiation. The agent appears to have a close similarity to the agent causing scrapie, and evidence shows that the disease arose in cattle after the feeding of animal protein containing nervous tissue from scrapie-infected sheep which had been insufficiently sterilised. Animals so infected would have received massive doses of the infectious agent.

In the UK all suspicious cases in cattle are slaughtered after confirmation. The evidence is that there is very little vertical transmission from cow to calf and reported cases are now falling very significantly. No animal protein is fed to ruminants, and the brain and spinal cord are removed from beasts at the slaughterhouse and destroyed. Thus there is reasonable hope that the disease in cattle will be eliminated. Fears that BSE may be transmitted to man are not justified by the evidence. (See Chapter 4 for a full description of BSE.)

Bloat

Bloat, also known as blown, hoven or tympanitis, is a common disorder of the rumen or first stomach and is one of several problems largely occurring from grazing. The rumen becomes distended with gas and the pressure from this on the diaphragm may lead to the animal dying from asphyxia or shock. Two types of bloat occur: the first is where the gases separate from the contents of the lower part of the rumen and the second where the gases remain as small bubbles mixed with the contents in a foamy mass, giving rise to what is known as 'frothy bloat'.

Bloat most often occurs in the grazing of lush pastures which contain a high proportion of clover. It is likely to happen when the herbage is growing rapidly in the late spring or early summer but cases can occur throughout the whole of the grazing season and in some areas it has proved troublesome even where cattle are grazing on kale in the winter months. There are several possible explanations for this problem: it may be due to the fact that some kinds of herbage contain substances that may cause paralysis of the rumen muscles and of other organs concerned in the process of rumination; or it may be due to the fact that more gas is produced than can be got rid of by eructation. It has also been suggested that bloat can be due to the result of foaming in the rumen caused by saponin and protein substances obtained from plants. Starches and sugars may also play a part and between them they produce a foam of great stability in the rumen.

Symptoms are obvious: distension of the abdomen which is particularly pronounced on the left flank between the last rib and hip bone. The swelling spreads as the attack becomes more severe and eventually the whole abdomen is swollen. In the early stages and sub–acute form, bloat is characterised by the animal's unusual behaviour; it becomes uneasy, moves from one foot to another, swishes its tail and occasionally kicks at the abdomen. Breathing becomes very distressed and rapid. If the attack is a severe one, any movement intensifies the discomfort and so the animal stands quietly with legs wide apart. If relief is not given very quickly, death from suffocation or exhaustion can follow rapidly.

Control

It is advisable to summon a veterinary surgeon as soon as possible. If time allows, a stomach tube may be inserted into the rumen to allow the gas out. In acute cases the only remedy is to puncture the rumen on the left flank with the surgical apparatus, the trocar and cannula. In an emergency, where death seems imminent and specialised assistance is not available, the only course of action is to puncture the area with a short pointed knife with a blade which is at least 6 inches long – the blade being plunged into the middle of the swelling on the left side and twisted at right angles to the cut to assist the gas to escape.

Although this treatment will serve to give immediate relief, more treatment is required if the case is one of frothy bloat. Drenching with one of the substances known as silicones, or with an ounce of oil of turpentine in a pint of linseed oil, often helps in the less severe cases and some gentle exercising may help to relieve the pressure of the gas in the rumen. There are also a number of medicinal treatments available, such as avlinox, which is an ethylene oxide derivative of ricinoleic acid.

Prevention

A number of methods have been used to control bloat and in this way the incidence of the most serious cases can be reduced to negligible proportions. Efficient pasture management can help to avoid the trouble. After a pasture is closely grazed and then rested, the clover recovers more quickly than the grasses, so that when pastures are used intensively the clover becomes dominant in the sward. It is not yet possible to assess the proportion of grass to clover needed to avoid the risk of bloat but it is generally considered that if there is less than 50% of clover present it is usually safe. A variety of seed mixtures has been tried to provide a suitable balance between clover and grass; one which has given promising results contains tall fescue. After it has been closely grazed this species of grass recovers almost as quickly as the clover and maintains a reasonably safe balance between grass and clover.

Another system which has been advocated is to allow the herd to graze a potentially dangerous herbage for a limited period and then turn it on to an old pasture for a time.

Controlled grazing can contribute to the prevention of bloat by ensuring that the grazing animal eats both leaf and stem, whether clover or grass, and that it cannot select clover or clover leaf which is thought to be the more dangerous. If an electric fence is moved forward so that the cows have access to a succession of narrow strips of pasture during the course of the day, bloat may be reduced or eliminated but it may reduce the intake of the feed and milk yield.

The second method of controlling grazing is to mow strips of herbage, then allow it to wilt and let the herd graze it as it lies on the ground. Alternatively, the wilted herbage can be carted to the cattle and fed indoors.

The feeding of roughage in the form of hay or oat straw shortly before the grazing of dangerous pasture has also been practised for many years. It is only completely reliable if the roughage is fed overnight.

It is also possible to feed anti-foaming agents, or even to spray the pasture with emulsified peanut oil. However, this is expensive and has to be done daily, so it is not a very practicable proposition.

Milk fever

Milk fever occurs in cows after calving, usually in dairy breeds of high milk-yielding capacity. It is given various synonyms, such as hypocalcaemia, parturient hypocalcaemia, parturient paresis and parturient apoplexy. There is, in fact, no fever and indeed it is more usual for the cows to show sub-normal temperatures.

Symptoms

The symptoms, which may not be noticed in the early stages, usually occur within 12–72 hours of calving, although occasionally they occur before calving and, in a few other cases, even months after calving. In its typical form, there is a short period of uneasiness with paddling of the hind legs, swishing of the tail and convulsive movements, but this is soon followed by depressed consciousness and paralysis. The animal usually falls on its side with its legs extended, rolling its eyes and breathing heavily. The characteristic picture is a twisting of the neck as it lies on one side, with spasm of the neck muscles, shallow laboured breathing, grunting, cessation of rumination and dryness of the muzzle. Bloat may occur and there is likely to be constipation. Other side effects can be pneumonia, inflammation of the uterus (metritis), retained afterbirth and strained tendons and muscles. In straightforward milk fever, the calcium and phosphorus levels fall and the magnesium levels rise.

In practice it is quite difficult to distinguish between the simple hypocalcaemia and the more complicated metabolic disorder where there are a number of deficiencies which have to be corrected.

The background to occurrence

There does not appear to be any real breed incidence, but it is usually well-fed, high-yielding cows which are affected and the severity of the condition increases with age: it is very rare at the first calving but after one attack it is more likely to occur at future calvings. The cause is usually ascribed to a temporary failure in the physiological mechanism which controls calcium levels in the blood. The stress of calving and the physical adjustment necessary for lactation will upset the balance of chemical regulators (hormones) produced by various glands and if the cow does not adjust itself quickly enough it may suffer an attack of parturient hypocalcaemia. The sudden fall in the level of calcium in the blood is not due to any shortage of calcium in the food and cannot be prevented by feeding extra calcium compounds, although it is of course essential that adequate calcium is always present.

Control

The immediate administration of a solution of calcium – calcium borogluconate is normally used – is highly effective in curing uncomplicated milk fever. It may be given intravenously for a quick response, or subcutaneously for a slower effect. If the case is recognised earlier, the latter is usually effective and may be given by the stockman. Where a more immediate effect is required the solution must be given by the intravenous route.

In addition to the administration of calcium, the cow should be propped up in the box by means of straw bales on each side to prevent it from becoming 'blown', and to prevent regurgitation of ruminant contents.

Further injection of calcium may be required and, in complicated cases, there will also be a need to administer phosphorus injections and even other materials. Professional advice is certainly required for all but the most simple case of hypocalcaemia.

One method frequently used in an attempt to prevent milk fever is to give the cow injections of Vitamin D. This vitamin increases the mobilisation of calcium in the body and may thereby help to prevent levels falling too low.

Ketosis (acetonaemia)

Ketosis is a disease involving ketones which are chemical compounds which may be produced during the metabolism of fat. This condition may occur when an animal's food intake is inadequate for its needs and it is drawing on its own reserves in considerable amounts to make good the deficiency. The usual form of ketosis is ketonaemia which includes an excess of ketones in the blood. Since acetone is the simplest and most characteristic of the ketones the disease is generally termed acetonaemia. It is also called 'post-parturient dyspepsia', as it often occurs soon after calving and is associated with indigestion. It often follows mild attacks of milk fever and almost appears to be an abnormally slow recovery, hence the traditional term for the disease of 'slow fever'.

Symptoms

The symptoms of ketosis are usually seen within 2 weeks of calving and in well-nourished stock of high milking capacity but it may also occur much later than this, even several months after calving. Ketosis is most common during the tail-end of winter. In the mild form it may almost pass unnoticed and be over within a few days, but it is readily recognised in its more severe forms. The cow will appear listless, with a marked loss of condition, dull coat and a sickly sweet smell of acetone in the breath and also in the urine and milk. The milk production falls away quickly and the milk becomes tainted and undrinkable. There is also a failure to co-ordinate muscles and the affected cow will find it difficult to walk straight so that it tends to stand in one position with its back arched and with straightened hocks. Constipation with dark, mucus-covered dung is usual. The pulse is variable and the temperature is usually either normal or slightly down. Sometimes there is a licking mania, a rather wild-looking appearance, champing of the jaws and salivation and there may also be hyper-excitability.

The condition is rarely fatal but it may become chronic and resistant to treatment. Chronic acetonaemia can last for months, during which time the milk will be unsaleable and the animal's condition will deteriorate to such an extent that the only economic action to take is to cull it from the herd.

Control

First, tests are carried out to confirm the presence of ketones in the blood. Usually the blood sugar will be low and glucose injections are an early response. Corticosteroids may be administered to give a longer-term beneficial effect. Other useful treatments are glycerine and preparations containing sodium propionate, molasses and/or molassine meal are also helpful.

Prevention will depend principally on skilful management. The energy provided in the food must keep pace with the draining demands of production, especially in early lactation. However, it is important not to increase concentrates too drastically or the cow may be put off them just when she needs them. In late pregnancy the cow should be kept in good condition but not over-fat. No excessive steaming-up is called for. The roughage in the ration should also be carefully selected and kept up to a good level or at least reduced slowly if the cow's appetite and enthusiasm for a balanced diet are to be maintained. Silage feeding can be a contributory factor to ketosis due to the high level of butyric acid produced when fermenting conditions are right. All changes in feed should be gradual and carefully watched. If feeding is balanced in all items and a sufficiency is always given, there is a minimum chance of ketosis occurring.

Hypomagnesaemia

The amount of magnesium in the blood of normal animals keeps within a fairly constant range. However, should the magnesium level of the blood drop below this range, then the condition known as hypomagnesaemia, or grass tetany, can result. The condition is widespread throughout the world but occurs especially in areas of cooler climate where the pasture has been improved and production increased. In adult cattle it is called by various names, such as 'grass tetany', 'grass staggers', 'lactation tetany' and 'Hereford disease', whilst in calves it is known as 'milk tetany' or 'calf tetany'.

The underlying causes

Possibly the main period of occurrence of this disease is in the period of sudden change for lactating cows from winter-housed conditions to those of the rapidly sown spring grass. However, although the occurrence of hypomagnesaemia does seem to be at its peak during the spring flush, and the autumn one to a lesser extent, it is now known to occur in cattle under most feeding and management regimes, including winter feeding periods. For all these reasons it seems fairly certain that the condition occurs in cattle on pasture which has a very adequate magnesium content. Underfeeding appears to be a predisposing cause, especially in out-wintered beef cattle, but overall the disease seems to be due to physiological dysfunctioning that interferes with the absorption and utilisation of the magnesium which is in the food and causes sudden falls in blood magnesium levels.

Symptoms

Symptoms vary according to the intensity of the attack. The first signs are often nervousness, restlessness, loss of appetite, twitching of the muscles, especially of the face and eyes, grinding of the teeth and, quite soon after, staggering. In less acute cases animals which are normally placid become nervous or even fierce. In severe cases paralysis and convulsions develop very soon after the onset of symptoms and if treatment is not given death will follow very quickly. In milking cows a sudden reduction in milk yield may occur just before an attack. Sometimes the attack comes on so rapidly that no symptoms are seen – merely a dead beast.

Hypomagnesaemia often starts at milking times or during feeding when the animals are more excited or disturbed. There is also a chronic form of the disease in which cows show a gradual loss of condition, although appetite and even the milk yield do not show any drop. This chronic state can last several weeks and then develop into the more acute condition.

In some cases where beef cattle are kept out all the year round, often without any shelter and under poor conditions, their blood magnesium levels 'cycle' in a regular seasonal way, being normal in summer, falling slowly in late autumn and winter, reaching a 'low' in early spring and then rising again to normal. In these cases there may be no clinical signs of abnormality but they can occur when calving or some other severe stress occurs during the periods of lower blood magnesium.

Hypomagnesaemia will sometimes occur at the same time as hypo-calcaemia or acetonaemia. Obviously in these cases the symptoms will be more complicated, with some signs of all the diseases, and only a blood examination will give the full picture.

Control

The moment signs are seen or suspected, veterinary advice should be sought. The veterinary surgeon may inject magnesium plus other solutions but it needs to be done by a qualified person for favourable results: haphazard use may kill the animal. Important measures need to be taken in an attempt to prevent the disease occurring. In most cases supplements of magnesium will prevent the condition. Two ounces of magnesium oxide per head per day have been used for many years successfully in dosing adults to prevent the condition. The magnesium oxide is usually given as calcined magnesite in a granular form; this must be given daily to cattle under risk or blood magnesium levels can fall quickly.

Although it is thought that the disease is not caused by a shortage of magnesium in the diet, the use on pastures of magnesium-rich fertilisers has been quite successful in preventing the disease. On some soils, top dressing in January or February with 500 kg of calcined magnesite per acre can be a perfect preventative, even 250 kg may be sufficient. Another method of preventing the disease is the magnesium 'bullet' in the reticulum with its slow release of magnesium and attempts have also been made to give multivitamin injections to increase the absorption and utilisation of magnesium. Such measures certainly help in preventing the disease but cannot replace the earlier methods given.

In out-wintered cattle where the condition occurs the incidence is highest during the coldest weather.

There appears to be no definite association with soil-type, nevertheless the condition does occur much more on some farms than others. It has been shown that the liberal use of nitrogen and potash fertilisers, especially on young leys, may increase the incidence of hypomagnesaemia but this also is by no means the whole story, since the condition occurs not infrequently on old and new pastures at various stages of growth and after treatment with a variety of different fertilisers.

The condition occurs in all breeds but is very uncommon in Jersey cows. In contrast to milk fever, hypomagnesaemia is not particularly associated with cattle giving high yields and it occurs as frequently in beef cattle as dairy cattle.

Calf tetany

Many years ago it was established that calves could not be reared to maturity on milk alone because of the onset of deficiency conditions and in particular hypomagnesaemia or calf tetany during growth. However, the condition also occurs under other conditions of feeding and it is an increasing problem in beef calves, especially if they are grazing at the time of the most active growth of spring grass.

The symptoms in calves are similar to those in older animals: hyperexcitability, irritableness and twitching of the muscle. The walk often becomes spastic, the feet being carried well above the usual height. As the disease progresses convulsions may follow and eventually death. Symptoms rarely occur before about 6 weeks of age and are often missed at first so that only the terminal convulsions are seen.

Treatment consists of immediate administration of suitable magnesium injections. Prevention is effected by administering about 15 g ($\frac{1}{2}$ oz) of calcined magnesite daily, or 30 g (1 oz) of magnesium carbonate daily.

Production diseases and the metabolic profile test

High production in dairy cattle is being achieved in two principal ways: first by intensification and improvement of management and feeding and, second, by selecting and breeding animals which give the highest milk yields. Both trends have inherent dangers in that the animals may fail to withstand the combined strain of high production under the most intensive conditions. All production systems have three parts:

(1)   An input of the raw material – the feed
(2)   An output of the finished product – in dairy cattle the milk
(3)   A processing system within the animal which is in fact extremely complex and under great strain in the high-producing animal

The problem of production disease occurs when input rates fail to keep pace with the output rates, or when the processing system in the middle becomes overloaded. When the dairy cow is confronted with an input/output imbalance she tends to use her own tissues to make good the deficiency and will 'milk herself into the churn'. The cow can use up so much of her vital reserves of materials that she can kill herself in an effort to maintain production.

Two types of metabolic disease can be distinguished. The first are those where there are very sudden and severe demands on a cow which she fails to meet: for example, at the birth of her calf. The flow of milk demands a surge of energy requirements and food will be insufficient for this at once so the cow draws on her reserves. If too much is taken a condition such as hypocalcaemia develops because the high level of calcium in the milk seriously reduces the calcium in the blood. The more chronic metabolic disease occurs when there is a gradual depletion of the reserves over a lengthy period. The best example is when the dairy cow gradually depletes her reserves with a high output of milk and marginally inadequate feed intake. Calcium and phosphorus will be drained from the skeleton, leading to the so-called 'broken down cow'. Ketosis is another major problem, due to insufficient carbohydrate for high production. The cow has to metabolise her body fat to make good the deficiency but if this goes too far there is collapse of carbohydrate metabolism followed by ketosis.

Another problem of a chronic nature is that due to trace element deficiency. Many pastures are deficient, for example, in iodine, sodium, manganese and copper.

Prevention of production diseases depends on balancing intake with output. Calculations based on a simple knowledge of the composition of the diet are not always sufficiently accurate. For instance, the maintenance part of the diet is impossible to assess with any great accuracy. If the cows are at pasture and even on indoor rations, analyses of hay and silage can be misleading and the cows may not be consuming all their share of the food supplied. Some kind of measure of the state of balance within the cows themselves is needed: a test to show the nutritional and metabolic status of a dairy herd. One test which gives a warning of an impending metabolic disease is the Compton Metabolic Profile Test; it is based on the blood chemistry of 21 cows whatever the size of the herd. Automatic analyses enable results to be obtained almost instantly. Tests for the following are usually done:

Protein	Magnesium
Albumin	Copper
Globulin	Sodium
Glucose	Potassium
Urea	Haemoglobin
Phosphate	Packed cell volume
Calcium	

Samples are taken from seven cows in each of the following groups:

❑ Cows on high production
❑ Cows whose yield has dropped a good deal
❑ Dry cows

Thus there is a total of 252 tests per herd.

The results throw light on causes of poor production or poor health, or indicate pointers to improvements in management or diet. They also show items of wastage in the diet so that appropriate action can lead to economies.

Mastitis

Mastitis literally means inflammation of the mammary gland or udder. It is, however, a term which is applied to all 'diseases' of the udder; most of these are caused by infectious agents of which there are a large number. Mastitis has always been an important disease of dairy cattle with potentially disastrous consequences but with the advent of antibiotic treatments there was a general optimism that the days of the disease were numbered; regrettably this has not been the case, for a number of reasons. Organisms that cause mastitis have become increasingly resistant to the constant use, or perhaps more correctly misuse and abuse, of antibiotic therapy. Even with the introduction of an ever-increasing range of antibiotics the agents causing the disease have tended to outstrip the medicines available.

Also there has been a growth of large dairy cattle units with greater opportunity for disease build-up and cross infection. Cow cleanliness has become less satisfactory and some of the most recent husbandry practices, for example loose housing and cubicles, lead to dirtier cows and udders. There has also been the emergence of different forms of mastitis, called environ-mental mastititis, because of their association with the newer forms of husbandry and rather different balance of organisms involved.

Thus a very worrying picture is presented that mastitis in the dairy cow may affect as many as 50% of the cows in the National Herd in one form or another, many causes being subclinical and so not readily recognisable. Since a cow with mastitis may *readily* lose a quarter of her milk output there is no doubt over the extreme economic importance of this condition. Whenever mastitis occurs it must be looked upon as a herd problem rather than a 'one-off' event and should be dealt with urgently and thoroughly. Even a single cow may be a warning of a management error and should be carefully considered in this respect.

Subclinical mastitis means that the udder is affected with a relatively mild bout of disease but it is not so apparent that the cow's health or even the milk yield is obviously affected. How can one know if this is the case? Diagnosis can now be done most efficiently by cell counts. If an inflammatory process is proceeding, the milk will contain more white blood cells than normal. The best way for the farmer to deal with this is to arrange for regular monitoring of the cells in the milk. The range of 'counts', with the sig-nificance given, is shown in Table 5.6.

The cell count tests are an excellent procedure as they can act as warnings and enable preventive measures to be implemented.

Table 5.6 Diagnosing subclinical mastitis from cell counts.

Cell count ranges (cells/ml)	Estimate of mastitis incidence in a herd	Estimate of milk (litres) production loss per cow
Below 250 000	Neglible	—
250 000–499 000	Slight	200 litres
500 000–749 000	Average	350
750 000–999 000	Bad	720
1 000 000 and over	Very bad	900

The milking machine

A major predisposing cause of mastitis is the misapplication of machine milking together with bad maintenance and a poor hygiene routine during milking.

One of the most serious of these is overmilking, i.e. the milking machine is left on much longer than it should be. There has long been a belief that it is critically necessary to extract the very last drop of milk. In many cases, too, the cowman has too much to do to give proper attention to each cow, so that he is totally overstretched. Overmilking tends to cause considerable damage to the very delicate mucous membranes lining the teat canal (Fig. 5.10) and this then allows pathogenic microorganisms to invade so that mastitis results. The cowman must see when the main flow of milk has stopped, then apply a mild pressure on the cluster to prevent it 'rising up' or enormous damage may be done since the force of the vacuum will grip the teat and a portion of membrane of the cistern is sucked into it forming an obstruction so that the milk cannot flow. The cowman may either machine-strip the udder of milk by holding the cluster down for 15 seconds or so, or the remaining milk may be left in the udder. Either course is perfectly acceptable, but leaving the machine on for too long is disastrous.

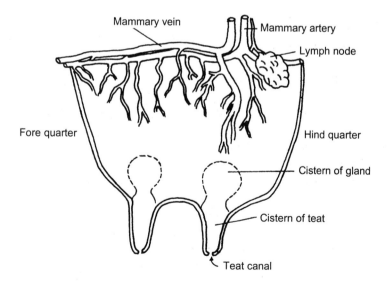

Fig. 5.10   Diagrammatic cross-section of a cow's udder.

Other items in connection with machine milking have an important bearing on mastitis. Teat liners of the right size and of gentle fit must be chosen, they must never be slack and should be carefully maintained to prevent them from causing damage. Pulsations of the machine must be maintained between 40 and 60 a minute; if the rate increases squeezing may fail and mastitis is more likely to occur. The ratio between the release and squeeze phase should be between 2:1 and 1:1.

There are other vital parts and procedures. The pump needs to be maintained properly as it 'ages' or a surge of milk may result around the teat, such circumstances also being a predisposing cause of mastitis. The vacuum regulator prevents fluctuation in vacuum which can be very damaging to the udder and teats for, if it fails, a surge of milk results around the teat and clusters may fall off or, if it rises, it damages the teats, causing extrusion of the lining of the teat canal.

No words here can overemphasise the importance of having regular expert maintenance of the milking machine. A very substantial number of machines on farms are faulty in one respect or another and can take a large share of the blame in causing mastitis.

Types of mastitis

There are various ways of classifying mastitis. It may be done on the basis of the *cause*, e.g. the type of bacteria or other pathogenic organisms that have invaded the udder, or it may be done on the basis of the *symptoms* of the disease. In the recognition and treatment of the disease both aspects are important.

The symptoms are probably the best starting point. There are easily recognisable forms of clinical mastitis. In this category are the *acute, sub-acute* and *chronic* forms.

Acute mastitis

The cow is obviously ill – feverish, fast-breathing, depressed and there is no cudding. Examination of the udder will show that one or more quarters are tense, swollen and possibly discoloured (blue); the cow will usually object strongly to the examination due to the severe pain. It may be possible to withdraw from the affected quarter(s) a small quantity of fluid, looking not so much like milk but more akin to a yellow serum, or perhaps containing blood with a pus-like, foul-smelling exudate. In such cases gangrene of the udder may set in very quickly, in effect causing the destruction of part of the udder around the base of the teat. This 'acute' mastitis, as it is clinically called, is often the same thing as the so-called 'summer mastitis' which, whilst it is most common in dry cows and heifers in the summer months, can occur in cows at other times. Such mastitis is caused primarily by a bacterium, *Corynebacterium pyogenes*, and may be treated with antibiotics and sulphur drugs. It is essential to treat acute mastitis early if there is any hope of retaining the cow's milking ability, although this is never very likely in any case. Because of its common association with 'dry cows' its incidence *may* be reduced by using long-acting antibiotic therapy as soon as the cow is dried off.

Sub-acute mastitis

The symptoms are somewhat similar to acute mastitis but milder and slower in their progress. The first sign of disease may be the appearance of small clots in the milk with some increased difficulty in extracting it. Pain also gradually increases and the affected quarter(s) swell. The milk eventually becomes yellowish and decreases in quantity. The cow does not usually become more than slightly ill, which clearly distinguishes it from the acute form.

Chronic mastitis

In this form of mastitis there is no pain, and any general sickness in the cow is unlikely, but there is a gradual hardening of the udder tissue, a decrease in the amount of milk and a progressive swelling of those quarters infected.

Causes of mastitis

At one time the most frequently occurring bacterium was *Streptococcus agalactiae*, but this has generally decreased in incidence with the advent of successful antibiotic treatment. Other streptococci, *S. dysgalactia* and *S. uberis*, are common as are staphylococcus and corynebacterium. There are, however, some serious new forms of mastitis that are of comparatively recent origin and are the most difficult to treat.

Escherichia coli is usually associated with so-called environmental mastitis. Pseudomonas is also a common bacterial cause of mastitis, as is *Corynebacterium bovis*. Mastitis may also be caused by microorganisms other than bacteria, such as mycoplasma (*M. agalactiae*) and moulds, the latter being termed mycotic mastitis.

Control of mastitis

It is now accepted that it is never going to be possible to eliminate mastitis by antibiotic treatment alone. This is because many preparations are not active against certain of the bacteria causing mastitis and also because so much infection remains subclinical and cannot therefore be recognised. Thus the view is now taken that the control of mastitis must depend largely on the application of hygienic procedures of the highest standard and these methods will now be discussed. Table 5.7 also sets out a summary of preventive measures against mastitis.

Table 5.7   A summary of measures aimed to prevent mastitis in the dairy cow.

❑ Basic design of cow accommodation must be right to ensure that the cow's bed is dry and clean and that there is a minimum chance of injury to the udder
❑ Replace fouled bedding frequently in stalls, yard or cubicles
❑ Test milking machine regularly, check vacuum pressures, pulsation rates, air bleeds and liners daily
❑ Monitor cell counts in milk. Keep detailed records for frequent reference
❑ Teat-dip always to be used after milking. Use a sanitising mixture with an emollient such as lanolin
❑ Wash udders before milking with clean running water and dry with disposable towels. Milker should preferably wear smooth rubber gloves
❑ Ensure early diagnosis by use of 'fore-milk' cup
❑ Treat all cases of mastitis promptly
❑ Cull chronic cases of mastitis
❑ Correct laboratory diagnosis of causal organisms assists in taking proper remedial measures
❑ Treat cows as they dry off with a long-acting antibiotic

Teat dipping
After milking, all teats should be dipped in antiseptic; this is usually based on an iodophor or chlorine solution which will not harm the tissue of the teat.

Cowman's hygiene
The cowman should wear smooth rubber gloves which can be dipped in the antiseptic before use.

Udder cleanliness
This is preferably achieved by using warm water sprays and then drying with disposable paper towels, which are much more effective than cloths which can cause cross-infection. If warm water cannot be used, cold water should be used first and then a good proprietary udder wash.

Good technique and equipment
The importance of this has already been fully emphasised.

Strip-cup
The routine use of the strip-cup where required is advisable. This device enables a little milk to be looked at from an udder and thus recognise the earliest appearance of mastitis.

Routine therapy
There is a vogue for the routine use of long-acting antibiotic intra-mammary treatments when cows are dried off. This is intended to get rid of any residual infection in the udder and also ensure that the cow does not have

any infection when it calves down again. The theory is good but very careful professional advice on what should and should not be done is necessary; such routine use of antibiotics is liable to cause drug resistance.

Culling

Careful consideration should be given to culling from the herd all those cows which are a constant source of mastitis.

Treatment with antibiotics

Clinical cases need prompt treatment but measures should be taken to ensure the use of the correct antibiotic. As a routine, when a case occurs a sample of milk should go to the laboratory *before* any treatment is instituted. Treatment does not have to wait until after the report is back but it will enable confirmation that it is the right antibiotic. If the antibiotic used is insensitive the necessary change can be made quickly. It is also worth emphasising that the course of treatment must continue for the full time advised, usually 5 days. One of the most serious errors of all is to administer the antibiotic for an insufficient period: this is one of the certain ways of producing resistant organisms.

Disease problems associated with breeding in cattle

Lowered fertility results in lowered production and causes great economic loss. However, infertility is not a disease as such, it is only the symptom of one. It may be due to any condition that prevents a vigorous sperm from fertilising a healthy ovum to produce a robust calf. The process involved is complicated and the different causes of infertility are numerous. Consider the whole physiological process. The bull must produce healthy sperm only, but the cow must not only produce a healthy egg but also provide the ideal condition for the fertilisation of the ovum by the sperm and the establishment of the embryo in the uterus. The cow then has to provide the nutrients for the calf and then, when it is mature, she must expel the calf from the uterus.

Infertility has probably become more serious in recent years because it tends to be associated with cows giving an immensely good yield of milk.

Causes of infertility

Fundamentally the breeding potential of an animal depends on certain inherited genetic tendencies and the presence of any inherited abnormalities. Such genes may either cause the animals to be infertile or produce faulty calves. However, some of the most important causes of infertility are bacterial or other infectious agents. Such an agent may be a specific organism producing a condition of which infertility is only one symptom. An example of this is contagious abortion (brucellosis), which is fully dealt with later in this chapter.

Another example is trichomoniasis, the causal organism being *Trichomonas foetus*, which is spread at service by infected bulls, which themselves show no obvious evidence of infection. A third example, vibriosis, is due to the organism *Vibrio foetus* and is carried and transmitted by apparently normal bulls. Both trichomonas and vibrio organisms multiply in the uterus and cause the death and abortion of the fetus. Infertility may also be caused by non-specific infections of the genital tract.

Control

When a cow or heifer fails to conceive to a second service it should be examined by a veterinary surgeon who, by carrying out tests, can establish if there is an infectious cause. If there is, it may well be treatable. Prevention depends on a number of factors. The herd should be kept as self-contained as possible and only maiden heifers and unused bulls should come into the herd. There should be no exchange of breeding animals. The diet must be adequate and balanced.

Trichomoniasis

Trichomoniasis is a veneral disease which is spread by bulls. It can be one of the most important causes of infertility in cattle and has from time to time caused serious losses to herds. Fortunately with the introduction and general adoption of artificial insemination in cattle the opportunity of cross-infection has greatly diminished.

The infective agent of trichomoniasis is a small microscopic parasite called *Trichomonas foetus*. The bull becomes infected from an infected cow and the parasites live in the crevices of the moist skin covering the penis. When an infected bull serves a heifer or cow the parasites pass into the female tract, where they are able to multiply. Once infected, the bull may transmit the infection to all the females he serves for the rest of his life. The disease is exclusively venereal and this is the only way it can spread, i.e. via the genitalia. Infected cows cannot infect non-infected females and all danger of infection is removed when the infected bull is removed.

The first symptom of trichomoniasis is usually a period of unsatisfactory breeding. The presence of the parasites in the uterus interfere with the progress of normal pregnancy and cows and heifers usually fail to hold to service and abortion will also occur.

There may be no other signs of infection and the disease may not be suspected for some time. Some small aborts may be seen from time to time; usually the abortions occur very early so they may be not seen and it may be thought the animals have merely failed to hold to service. Sometimes a discharge occurs after the infection is established. Thus a suspicion of infection would be aroused when a number of animals fail to hold to repeated service and especially if the interval is in the period of 2–4 months.

Diagnosis of infection is made on a laboratory test of mucus collected from a number of females or, in the case of the bull which probably shows no symptoms, the parasites can be found in washings from the prepuce of the bull.

Control of this infection is done in two principal ways. Firstly, the use of a bull should be abandoned at least temporarily and replaced by artificial insemination. No bull should be used again on a cow in an 'infected' herd until after a normal calf has been produced by artificial insemination. The infection of a bull is sufficiently permanent and resistant to treatment to recommend that infected bulls are culled from the herd.

It is clear that it is possible to eradicate the disease from a herd by appropriate management techniques. The foregoing advice also stresses the importance of having good records at one's disposal, since this is the only way the presence of a disease can be suspected early on, to achieve minimum loss and maximum results.

Vibriosis

Vibriosis is a disease affecting the genital organs of cattle which leads to infertility and abortion. The symptoms are rather similar to those of trichomoniasis. The condition is caused by a bacterium, *Vibrio foetus*, which is also a true venereal infection spread during service. A bull may contract the disease initially by mating with an infected heifer or cow, or indeed by contracting the infection in unhygienic quarters. Fortunately the disease is of rather low incidence but when it arises the effects can be very serious.

Infertility and abortion are the only obvious symptoms. Cows and heifers return to service at irregular intervals – some may return after several months – so the economic loss is particularly serious. After a period of infection in a herd, the condition may tend to become less serious and it is very important under the rather vague and variable conditions of the disease to have laboratory examinations in order to see that it is properly diagnosed.

Control is dependent on a number of different procedures. The herd is best divided into two groups – one being the males and females which have not been exposed to infection, and the other consisting of all the other breeding animals which are or may have been infected. This latter group remains as a possible cause of infection and should have separate arrangements for service. It is possible to treat infected bulls with antibiotics to eliminate the disease, although the safest way of stopping further infection is to use artificial insemination. This should enable elimination of infection altogether because the evidence suggests that cows clear the infection out after a pregnancy.

The following techniques to maintain freedom from infection also illustrate the general principles of preventing venereal diseases from being introduced into a herd:

❑ Only bulls which have never been mated, or have only been used with maiden heifers should be purchased
❑ It is best to obtain bulls only from herds which are known to be free of infection
❑ Females from other herds should never be brought into a herd for mating and only maiden heifers or cows from herds known to be free of disease should be brought in as replacements

Diseases affecting cattle of all ages

Foot-and-mouth disease

Foot-and-mouth disease is an acutely contagious disease which causes fever in cattle and all cloven-hoofed animals, followed by the development of blisters or vesicles, which arise chiefly on the mouth and feet. The disease is an infection, world-wide in incidence, caused by at least seven major variants of the foot-and-mouth virus. Each type produces the same symptoms and they can only be identified by specialist examination. The disease is notoriously contagious, perhaps more so than any other disease, it is known that it can spread as much as 50 miles downwind from one outbreak to another. It has a fairly short incubation period of about 3–6 days and can spread rapidly throughout a susceptible population.

The disease does not usually cause deaths, except in the young, but it leads to damaging after-effects: it will seriously lower productivity in all animals, especially the milking cows; mastitis will possibly develop so milk production is permanently impaired and the infection of the hooves may lead to lameness that leads to secondary infections.

Infection with the virus of foot-and-mouth disease can occur in many ways, other than by wind-borne spread. People, lorries, markets, wild birds and other animals, wildlife such as hedgehogs and so on are just some of the ways in which the disease can spread. In addition, infective material can come in from abroad in imported substances, such as hay, and meat and bones which have not been sterilised.

In this country foot-and-mouth disease is a notifiable disease and has long been dealt with by immediate slaughter of infected animals, this has been a very successful policy and has meant there have been few outbreaks. In fact, the last big outbreak occurred in 1967 and there have been just two small infections since then. The important thing is to be sure of recognising a case as soon as possible so all the official measures can be taken to control the disease. Symptoms that would lead one to suspect foot-and-mouth disease are described below.

Infected cows suffer from fever and anorexia with a sudden drop in milk yield and there are blisters on the upper surface of the tongue and the balls of the heels of the feet. There may be profuse, frothy slobbering to be seen around the mouth, and falling to the ground. There is also a sucking sound produced by partial opening of the mouth. All this starts very early on in the period of infection and so too does the evidence of pain in the feet. Animals prefer to lie down but when they are forced to walk they move painfully, occasionally shaking their feet. The lameness then becomes worse so the animal can barely move. Because the animals cannot eat and with all the resultant discomfort they soon lose weight and condition and often blisters develop on the teats so that the cow cannot be milked. Blisters are present in the early stages on the dental pad inside the lips and on the muzzle; the blisters start as small white vesicles containing fluid, then quickly enlarge to the size of a walnut. Several blisters may join together to form a very large one, they burst and leave a raw area underneath; much the same thing happens with the feet, leaving raw and sore areas.

The control of foot-and-mouth disease

The procedure in the UK, which is also used in many other countries, is to slaughter all the animals diagnosed as having the disease and all those in such close contact that they would almost certainly contract it. All examinations of the economics of the slaughter policy have shown it to be the least costly. The infected premises are then cleaned and disinfected and left empty for about 6 weeks before they can be restocked. Many restrictions are also imposed on the movement of susceptible animals within a 5–10 mile radius around the infected premises and no movement of animals is allowed out of this area. Restrictions, may, if necessary, be imposed on an even larger area. In the UK a legal provision has been made for limited use, if felt desirable, for the vaccination of a ring of stock around infected premises in an endeavour to stop virtually any spread at all. One should also be aware of obligations as a stock owner. If there is any suspicion that the animals have foot-and-mouth disease, then the police or a veterinary surgeon should be informed; they will take the official action required although the premises should be isolated in the meantime. No one who has been in contact with the stock should go amongst other animals. No animals, vehicles, feed, milk, etc., should be moved from the suspected premises and so far as possible no person should leave, nor should anything be taken on to the premises. Thus with all these precautions and many others that can officially be brought into action, there is the maximum chance that the outbreak will be contained.

In certain other countries where the disease is endemic, vaccines alone are used to control the disease.

Foot and mouth disease is still of enormous economic importance and there are currently outbreaks of great seriousness in the Far East, a particularly vicious outbreak occurring in 1995.

Rabies

Rabies is a notifiable virus disease which affects nearly all animals and is especially dangerous to man. It causes progressive paralysis and madness in most animals. The virus is present in the saliva so that the animals affected may bite one another, or man, and in this way cause infection to spread. It is nearly always fatal. The greatest danger represented by this disease is that infection becomes endemic – virtually permanent – in wild animals, particularly foxes but also in badgers, deer and vampire bats, and these infect dogs, cats and farm animals. Thus the particular danger to man is created.

The disease may be prevented in man and animals by vaccination, but it should be emphasised that no vaccinations are 100% effective and it is difficult to exaggerate the ghastly effects of this disease in humans. Nevertheless, the effectiveness of vaccines is constantly improving and it is likely that the use of vaccine as a control measure will increase.

One of the features of the virus is that after an animal becomes infected, perhaps via the saliva by being bitten by another rabid animal, several months may elapse before any signs of the disease are seen.

Symptoms

Symptoms in animals may show great variation, ranging from the classical mad, biting, salivating beast to 'dumb' forms in which the animals are incoordinate, progressively paralysed and make no noise. Usually the 'dumb' form follows the mad stage.

Control

The British Isles have been free of rabies outside quarantine for 75 years, other than two cases in dogs which were quickly dealt with. Our rigid regulations prohibiting the importation of dogs and cats and certain other mammals without a 6 month quarantine period which includes vaccination is thoroughly justified. The fear remains that animals incubating the disease may be smuggled in – or could jump off a boat – and thereby rabies could become endemic in the wild animal population. This danger has increased with the spread of rabies in areas of continental Europe near the UK. In those countries where the disease is endemic, great strides are now possible towards eradicating rabies with the aid of the greatly improved vaccines now available.

In the UK a House of Commons Select Committee recommended that the policy of quarantining dogs and cats on entry to this country be abandoned in favour of a vaccination procedure. This has not so far been put into place but it appears likely that this will happen within the near future.

Brucellosis

This is a specific contagious disease of cattle widespread throughout the work, caused principally by a bacterium, *Brucella abortus*, though some other species of this bacterium occur in cows and other livestock. It is also known as contagious abortion or Bang's disease. *Brucella melitensis* principally infects goats but also infects cattle, while *Brucella abortus suis* causes abortion in pigs but may also infect cattle.

Infectivity and symptoms

Fortunately the disease is now virtually eradicated in cattle in this country so the danger is removed. Because the way in which its eradication has taken place is so valuable as a lesson in disease control it is worth looking at this briefly. Brucellosis infects both the bull and the cow and the organism has a predilection for the reproductive organs. In the bull it affects the genitalia; in the cow it causes a chronic inflammation of the uterus and usually, but not by any means always, causes abortion of the fetus between the fifth and sixth month of pregnancy. Infected cows that do not abort may be carriers of organisms. Infected animals do become immune but they may be carriers for an uncertain and lengthy period.

After abortion, or after the calf is born at full term, there will be a period during which the animal excretes large numbers of the brucella organisms. These can then infect other animals by any route – via ingestion or via service, or by the stockman who handles infected material.

Control

There is no therapeutic cure for this condition that is effective enough to be advised. Control has therefore centred on testing for infected animals and slaughtering. In the meantime young stock are vaccinated with safe vaccines for a period of time and then, once the disease has been virtually eradicated, the vaccination can be stopped. However, testing must continue thereafter for a prolonged period.

Great Britain was declared free of brucellosis in cattle in 1981 and she joined, rather belatedly, several other European countries in virtually eliminating this condition. Other countries continue their efforts to the same end. Eradication is almost invariably achieved by a combination of agglutination and other testing procedures on sera and milk, the vaccination of young stock, usually with the Strain 19 vaccine, and slaughter of adult reactors. Such measures are combined with good hygiene procedures and need to be supervised by Government Veterinary Services backed by legally enforced regulations.

Tuberculosis in cattle

Tuberculosis is a chronic infectious disease affecting virtually all species of animals including man and birds and is due to a bacterium, *Mycobacterium tuberculosis*. There are three main strains of this organism. There is a strain which primarily affects humans but can also affect cattle; the cattle (bovine) strain which is most prevalent in cattle but also affects man, pigs and certain types of wildlife; and finally we must be aware of the avian strains which primarily affect birds but also cattle, pigs and other animals at times. All types of cattle may be affected but it is in the dairy cow that the main risk occurs. The milk from an infected dairy cow may contain the organisms that cause infection and this may affect calves or human subjects if the milk is not pasteurised or sterilised. Also, in advanced cases of tuberculosis, the uterus may become infected so that the calf is born with the disease.

Because the disease is usually chronic and the course of the disease slow it may be some time after the animal is infected that it shows any signs of the disease, but it is quite capable of causing infection in others long before this period occurs. Usually the first sign of disease is a lack of thrift and some progressive wasting of the animal. This will probably be accompanied by a cough – tuberculosis is essentially a disease of the lungs. In addition there may be an infection and hardening of the udder, and the milk that is produced contains tuberculous organisms and is thus highly dangerous. The milk may look quite normal until the later stages of the disease and eventually becomes watery and bluish in colour. Tuberculosis is essentially a slow, inflammatory action which produces almost anywhere in the organs of the body nodular swellings, known as tubercules, which are composed of fibrous tissue with a core of pus-like, caseous (cheesy) material.

Fortunately it is possible to test an animal for the presence of the disease long before it has reached the contagious stage. This is done by injecting a preparation known as tuberculin, made from tuberculous organisms. If an animal is infected this small injection of tuberculin into the skin of the animal will cause a reaction, but not when it is completely healthy. In fact, because the reaction could be due to a sensitivity to avian tuberculosis – and this is not a disease of any importance – an injection of avian tuberculin is also given and the difference between the two will be used to give the interpretation that is necessary. The conduct and interpretation of the test, known as the Intradermal Comparative Test, is a skilled operation and is conducted only by the veterinarian.

Tuberculosis has been virtually eradicated from the UK, although testing continues and some cases do occur. Recently there has been an increase in certain parts of the UK which is of real concern since the reason has not been established. Animals may be infected by man and wildlife: there is, for example, much concern about the infection of cattle by badgers which, in some areas, are serious reservoirs of the disease. Those same measures that have generally been successful in eliminating tuberculosis in the UK are also being applied in a similar fashion elsewhere.

It is worth noting that there is evidence that cows may be as much at risk of catching tuberculosis from humans as humans are from cows, a finding which is not unique to this disease.

Anthrax

Anthrax is a serious bacterial disease which infects cattle, other animals (see pig diseases) and man and tends to be fatal in both cattle and man. It is rare to see symptoms in cattle as infection is so acute that it usually causes sudden death. The cause of the disease is a bacterium, *Bacillus anthracis*, which once present, may persist in the soil of a farm, almost indefinitely. However, few cases occur in cattle in the UK because of the means taken to prevent its spread and re-infection. The means by which this is done are so important that attention will be drawn to each facet as a useful example of disease control methods.

Anthrax should be suspected if an animal is found dead or there is a very high fever and a large swollen neck; at either point professional help should be sought. Diagnosis is made by the veterinary surgeon by taking a very small quantity of blood and examining this under the microscope. If the animal dies from anthrax, or is infected with it, the blood would be teeming with the rod-shaped organisms that are distinctive features of this disease. *A major warning: do not allow the carcass to be cut or air to reach the blood since it is then that the organisms form spores which can survive for many years.* Some blood may be oozing from parts of the animal and this must be treated with disinfectant. Anthrax is a notifiable disease and measures that must be taken are mandatory. The carcass must be burned or buried deeply so that it is removed from any opportunity to cause re-infection, or for the organisms to form spores. The area around which the animal was found dead should be disinfected and isolated for a short while in case of spillage of the organisms. It is most likely that the source of infection is from a feedstuff – possibly meat or bone meal – which has come from imported infected material. Usually cases are isolated individual ones so it is not necessary to protect other animals but, if there is a risk, the animals can be given the hyperimmune antiserum or penicillin for immediate protection or relief, or longer-term protection by using a vaccine. Anthrax is much more common in hot countries, particularly in many parts of Africa where the climatic conditions favour its spread and where hygiene is noticeable by its absence.

Enzootic bovine leucosis (EBL)

This is a comparative newcomer to the list of notifiable diseases. It is a virus disease, slow and insidious in its effect, which may have been imported with Canadian Holstein cattle. It causes multiple tumours, known as lympho-sarcomas, and whilst it is certainly not widely present in the UK, its presence has been confirmed. The symptoms in the live and adult animal are chronic ill-health, anaemia, weakness and loss of appetite, which are not diagnostic. Only special laboratory examinations will give a definite diagnosis.

External parasites

Insects of various types (Fig. 5.11) which cause trouble to livestock in various ways – by frightening them, by irritation, biting, blood sucking, or by damage caused by the maggots (larvae) on the skin or flesh. All insects can also act as vectors of disease.

The warble fly

There are two species of cattle warble fly that cause trouble: *Hypoderma lineatum* and *Hypoderma bovis*. Both are rather like bumble bees in appearance as their dark bodies are covered in white, yellow and black hairs. They have

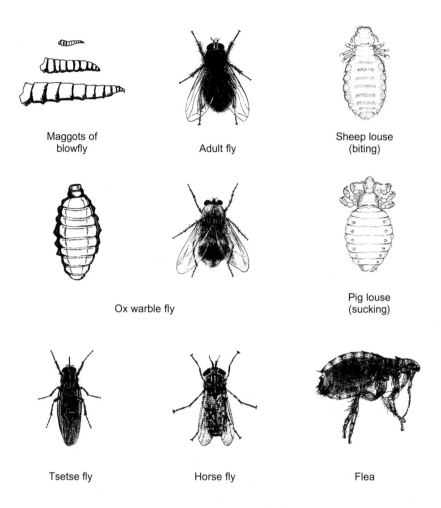

Maggots of blowfly

Adult fly

Sheep louse (biting)

Ox warble fly

Pig louse (sucking)

Tsetse fly

Horse fly

Flea

Fig. 5.11   Some insect pests that affect farm animals.

no mouths and only live for a few days. They are found almost everywhere in the British Isles and most other parts of the world.

Adult female flies cause substantial losses to cattlemen, being responsible for 'gadding'; this is the stampeding which results when cattle become worried and restless because of the presence of flies. Such stampeding lowers milk yield and may cause serious injuries to the beasts and even broken limbs. There is also hide damage, and this is by far the worst loss. The maggots of the fly make breathing holes and these can ruin parts of the hide. Even after the maggot has left the hide and the hole has healed over with fibrous tissue, it remains a weak area in the leather so that it has a much reduced value. The meat itself is also damaged: a yellowish jelly-like substance forms around each maggot and spoils the appearance of the meat.

The life cycle of the warble fly is as follows. During the short life of the fly the female may lay some 500 or so eggs which are attached to hairs on the legs and bellies of cattle, those of *H. bovis* being laid singly (like louse eggs) and those of *H. lineatum* in rows of up to about 20. In 4–5 days the eggs hatch and tiny maggots emerge, crawl down the hair and burrow through the skin of the beast by means of sharp mouth hooks.

The entry of the maggot causes some injury and it shows as a small pimple or scab. Under the skin the maggot moves along, feeding and growing. It takes 7–8 months to reach the skin of the animal's back. When this point is reached the maggots make breathing holes and become isolated within a small abscess. Each maggot stays there for 5–7 weeks, casting its skin twice and growing to a length of about 2.5 cm. The full-grown maggot is dark brown, fleshy, barrel-shaped and covered with groups of tiny spines. When fully ripe they squeeze themselves out of their 'warbles' and fall to the ground. Here they slide into shallow crevices in the soil or pass underneath dead vegetation. The skin of the maggot darkens and it then becomes a puparium or chrysalis, inside which the marble fly is formed. This usually takes about 4 weeks.

Control

Control must be achieved by dealing with the maggot. These can be destroyed by treating the animal with one of the more recently produced systemic insecticides.

Warble fly is a notifiable disease. The disease had been eradicated from the UK but has been reintroduced in recent years due to the importation of infected cattle, although no cases occurred during 1995 or 1996. Any suspicions must be reported to the divisional veterinary officer of the ministry who will supervise treatment of all cattle over 12 weeks old on the premises. Great care is needed in the use of the systemic insecticides as they are organophosphorus compounds and are administered by pouring on the backs of the animals or by injection. Sick animals must not be treated. Milking cows must be treated immediately after milking to allow at least 6 hours to elapse before the next milking. The approved 'withdrawal' period – which is on the label of the product used – will specify that no animal may be slaughtered for meat under 14–21 days after treatment.

Lice

Lice infestation is only a major problem in cattle when they are housed. The thick winter coat, lack of sufficient air and sunlight and possibly poor nutrition can contribute to the occurrence of this problem. Four species of lice infest cattle, three of which are sucking lice and the fourth, which is also the commonest, a biting louse. The sucking lice are *Haematopinus eyrysternus, Linognathus vituli* and *Solenoptes capillatus,* and the biting louse is *Damalinia bovis.* The sucking lice cause the greater damage and irritation as their sharp mouth parts pierce the skin to draw blood on which they feed. The biting louse, on the other hand, feeds on the scales of the skin and on the discharge from existing small wounds.

These four types of louse affect only cattle and cannot exist on other farm animals. The entire life-cycle takes place on the skin of the animals, where the females lay eggs on the skin in small groups which are attached to the base of the hair by a sticky secretion. There the eggs remain for up to 3 weeks, after which the young lice hatch out and very quickly start feeding and reproducing. Reproduction lasts for about 5 weeks; each female is able to lay about two dozen eggs and if conditions are favourable the number of lice can increase very rapidly. Lice cannot survive for more than 3–4 days away from cattle so transfer of infection is largely by direct contact.

It is not too difficult to recognise an infestation with lice. Lice tend to congregate on the animal's shoulders, the base of the neck, the head and the root of the tail. Examination of these areas will show them to be extremely scurfy and the lice should be obvious. As the infestation worsens more and more of the body can become affected. The affected animals rub and scratch themselves, greatly adding to the damage. The hair goes altogether in some areas. Rubbing thickens the skin which often breaks, so that bacterial infection gets in. A bad infestation will ultimately cause much loss of condition and production and should not be tolerated.

Insecticides must be applied to kill the lice, and materials that are satisfactory include organophosporus compounds, amitraz and synthetic pyrethroids. After treatment liquid preparations can be applied either under pressure or with a scrubbing brush. As these preparations have a reasonable residual effect, it is feasible for one good application to kill the lice and the larvae that hatch out after the application.

After treatment, measures must be taken to prevent reinfestation by contact with untreated animals and also by putting in fresh bedding and probably cleaning equipment. Never underestimate the damage that can be done by lice as a mechanical irritator and as vectors of any livestock disease.

Minerals and health

Cattle suffer from all the problems associated with minerals, that is, too little, too much, or the unavailability to the animal of a mineral which may be present in the feed in abundance. There are also problems with minerals being present in the ration in sufficient amounts but then for some reason accumulating within the animal body in an abnormal amount. Copper provides a good example of all of these features.

Copper

Copper is an essential element in the metabolism of livestock. Normally copper is present in herbage at a level between 7 and 25 parts per million of dry matter. If, however, the copper content of the grass falls below 5 ppm a copper deficiency may occur in animals grazing the pastures.

This simple type of copper deficiency is not common and it is much more likely for a 'conditioned' deficiency to be produced due to an excess of molybdenum in the pasture. An excess of molybdenum in the grass can lead to reduced copper storage in the liver, but this is not the only conditioning factor because copper deficiency may also occur on pastures of normal molybdenum content. It thus seems impossible to predict the possible copper status of animals from chemical examination of feeding stuffs or soils in this country except in the case of obviously 'teart' pastures which in the UK are especially common in Somerset.

Copper deficiency in soil is not confined to any particular soil type, although it tends to be more common in peaty areas.

Symptoms are rather indefinite and are not specific to this condition. The principal sign is a progressive loss of condition. The animals may scour badly; calves are more seriously affected than adults. The first signs of the disease may appear after the animals have been at grass for about a month; the calves appear stunted with their coats rough and discoloured. An almost diagnostic feature is that the hair round the eyes often changes colour or falls out, giving a spectacled appearance.

If copper deficiency is suspected then it is essential to have the blood analysed. If a deficiency is confirmed, copper can be administered as appropriate in the food or as a drench or by injection.

Copper poisoning is not uncommon in cattle. Only very small amounts are needed by cattle and poisoning usually occurs as a result of simple overdosing or overenthusiastic correction of a shortage.

Cobalt

Cobalt is another mineral that is needed in minute amounts by cattle and sheep and the common condition of 'pining' in sheep, due to a cobalt deficiency and fully described in Chapter 7, also affects cattle to a lesser but nevertheless significant degree. Deficiencies can cause unthriftiness, delayed puberty and infertility and occur in the UK in areas of the West Country,

Ireland and Scotland due to pasture deficiency but more especially in North America, Australia and South Africa.

Molybdenosis (teart)

Teart is the Somerset name for a scouring disease of cows and young cattle which has existed especially in certain local areas of that county. Such pastures are termed 'teart' as they produce the disease which is due to excessive amounts of the element molybdenum in the grass and soil. Pastures normally contain molybdenum at a level of 0.5–5.0 parts per million of the dry matter of the grass, at these levels there is no harm to the animals but on teart pastures the level of molybdenum rises up to 100 ppm and 20–40 ppm is very common. The chief areas of teart pastures are some 20 000 acres in Somerset but the problems do occur elsewhere. The severity of the disease depends essentially on the amount of soluble molybdenum in the herbage and this is at its maximum during periods of rapid growth in the spring. Symptoms shown, especially at this time, will include scour with yellow-green, evil-smelling dung. The animals become dirty, develop discoloured coats, lose condition rapidly and may eventually die.

The scour can be treated by the administration of copper supplements or injections. A daily amount of extra copper, about 1 g, is all that is required. This can be given conveniently in the form of anti-teart cake or copperised dairy cubes or, if preferred, by injecting a suitable copper preparation.

Lead poisoning

Lead poisoning is a very well known and documented condition but in spite of this the inherent dangers of old paints and other compounds containing lead are still not entirely appreciated. A large number of deaths still occur from this poison, especially in young calves, which tend to lick and chew all the fittings which in many cases may have residues of lead paint.

The symptoms of lead poisoning usually develop slowly. The first signs are dullness and loss of appetite, followed by signs of abdominal pain, grinding of the teeth, salivation and constipation. On other occasions there may be no symptoms at all until a few hours before death, when the animal abruptly starts bellowing, staggering and rolling eyes and frothing at the mouth before it collapses and dies. There are usually several intermittent convulsive phases during which the animal is very excitable and attempts to push against or climb walls. It appears to be blind and does not react to any outside stimulus but if the animal is not watched closely, these acute symptoms may be missed and it will be found dead because the phase of extreme excitation is often short.

Post–mortem signs may include inflammation of the abomasum and the adjoining few feet of the small intestine, or sometimes much further. Confirmation depends on the presence of abnormal amounts of lead in the liver and kidneys.

Lead poisoning usually arises from paint, woodwork, metal, tarpaulins, roofing felt, old paint tins and putty containing red or white lead: also old batteries and vegetation sprayed with lead arsenate. It is also possible for the calves to contract lead poisoning from lead derived from old lead pipes and cisterns. Lead poisoning is treated with magnesium preparations by the veterinary surgeon.

Table 5.8   The health of cattle: a summary of diseases, prevention and treatment.

Disease	Prevention	Treatment
Anthrax	(Notifiable in UK) Vaccine. Antiserum	Antiserum. Penicillin and broad-spectrum antibiotics
Blackquarter	Vaccine. Antiserum. Drain known infected land which is usually marshy	Antiserum. Amoxycillin or other broad-spectrum antibiotics
Bloat	Reduce intake of 'lush' material or other inciting food products	Deflate with stomach tube or needle. Silicones. 'Oil of turpentine'. Arachis oil. Antibiotics
Bovine spongiform encephalopathy (BSE or mad cow disease)	(Notifiable in UK) Do not feed animal protein that may contain infected material	None. Slaughter affected animals
Bovine viral diarrhoea (BVD)	Blood test and remove infected stock	None
Brucellosis	(Notifiable in UK) Vaccination. Removal of reactors. Improve hygiene	Slaughter of infected animals advisable. Otherwise use broad-spectrum antibiotics to assist recovery
Calf diphtheria	Disinfection of utensils and accommodation	Sulphonamides. Chlortetracycline. Oxytetracycline. Amoxycillin
Calf scour due primarily to *E. coli*	Colostrum. Regular and correct access to feed. Improve housing and hygiene	Warmth. Antiserum. Vaccine. Supportive fluid therapy. Broad-spectrum antibiotics, e.g. amoxycillin, tetracyclines
Coccidiosis	Cleanliness in rearing. Drain infected ground or remove cattle	Potentiated or other sulphur drugs
Foot-and-mouth disease	(Notifiable in UK) Vaccination if legally allowed	Usually slaughter infected animals and in-contacts. Antibiotic therapy assists

Table 5.8 Continued

Disease	Prevention	Treatment
Husk	Use only clean and well-drained land. Vaccine	Doramectin. Ivermectin. Levamisole. Oxfendazole
Hypomagnesaemia	Magnesium application to pasture or magnesium dosing or 'bullets'	Intravenous magnesium solution
Ketosis	Improve nutrition	Inject glucose solutions. Sodium propionate. Corticosteroids. Glycerine. Molasses
Lice	Improvement of hygiene and husbandry	Organophosphorus compounds. Amitraz. Synthetic pyrethroids
Liver fluke	Avoid marshy land. Kill secondary hosts (snails) on pasture with chemicals	Oxyclozanide. Nitroxynil. Albendazole. Rafoxanide
Mange	Improve hygienic procedures around buildings and remove infected animals	Amitraz. Ivermectin. Organophosphorus compounds. Synthetic pyrethroids
Mastitis	Attend to milking procedures, equipment, housing and hygiene. Antibiotics as appropriate to infection	Antibiotics via teat, single or in combination. Sensitivity to be verified
Milk fever	Improve nutrition. Inject Vitamin D	Inject calcium borogluconate and Vitamin D and consider other mineral needs such as magnesium and phosphorus by injection
Navell-ill (joint-ill)	Improve hygiene. Dress navel with antiseptics	Broad-spectrum antibiotics, e.g. amoxycillin, chlortetracycline, oxytetracycline
Parasitic gastroenteritis	Revise husbandry methods to prevent infestation and its effects	Doramectin. Ivermectin. Benzimiadoles. Levamisole
Rabies	(Notifiable in UK) Vaccination	Slaughter all infected animals
Redwater	Vaccines. Imizal. Acoprin. Diampron. Gonacrine	Use drugs listed under Prevention

Table 5.8   Continued

Disease	Prevention	Treatment
Respiratory disease of cattle	Improve environment, especially ventilation. Increase space. Separate different ages. Judicious use of antiserum and vaccines	Broad-spectrum antibiotics, e.g. amoxycillin, chlortetracycline. Sulphonamide
Ringworm	Clean buildings, separate infected stock	Local application of e.g. formalin, imidazole or systemic treatment with griseofulvin or sodium iodide
Salmonellosis	(Notifiable under Zoonoses Order in UK) Check feed to ensure freedom from salmonella. Check possibility of 'carriers'. Destroy rodents. Vaccine	Isolation. Amoxycillin and other antibiotics. Supportive fluid therapy
Tuberculosis	(Notifiable in UK) Test for reactors and slaughter	Usually none as infected animals should be removed and slaughtered
Warble fly	(Notifiable in UK) Systemic organophosphorus compounds, e.g. crufomate, trichlorphon	As Prevention
Wooden tongue and lumpy jaw	Disinfection and improved hygiene	Streptomycin. Iodides. Broad-spectrum antibiotics

Chapter 6

The Health of Pigs

As with most farm animals, there have been great changes in husbandry methods and the type of diseases in recent years. The well-known, traditional scourges of pigs, such as swine fever, foot-and-mouth disease and paratyphoid, have been eliminated in many countries or have been very well controlled. Instead, we are faced with extremely irksome, debilitating infections of the respiratory and enteric systems that are very difficult to eliminate entirely although it is possible by applying rigid standards of hygiene and management.

At present in pig husbandry there is a great dependence on 'background' medication, usually given via the feed, which is costly and never entirely satisfactory. Husbandry systems have developed without very much thought being given to disease control and the elimination of straw or other bedding in many modern systems. Improving the efficiency of muck handling has often caused welfare and additional disease problems and even a serious nuisance problem to the local population because of offensive smells, nausea and enteritis.

Diseases of pigs are dealt with here on the same basis as the other livestock, considering the diseases on a life-cycle basis, starting with those diseases affecting the sow and piglet around farrowing and then tracing through the ages of the pig to maturity and into the breeding period. Sadly, in some ways, few pigs continue in a herd for long so that there are remarkably few pigs on the farm that may be deemed fully mature.

The health of the sow and piglet around farrowing

Losses in young piglets are considerable: 10% of those born alive die within the first few days of life.

Some years ago, when surveys indicated that losses were averaging about 20%, it was established that some 50% of these were due to 'mechanical' or physical causes. A high proportion of piglets died from cold and another high percentage from crushing by the sow when she lay on the piglets. The first problem has very largely been eliminated by providing heated nests, and the crushing has been greatly reduced by providing various types of farrowing crates. However, in spite of this, losses, now largely due to disease, remain surprisingly high.

The underlying cause of the resurgence of disease in young piglets is probably due to the increased concentration and size of units combined with an often pitiful neglect of hygiene in the maternity area. The fundamental importance of an 'all-in, all-out' policy for the farrowing unit cannot be emphasised too strongly and allied to this should be a rigid disinfection of the building and cleaning of the sow herself, who often comes in dirty from the previous housing. Figure 6.1 shows an example of hygienically excellent farrowing accommodation.

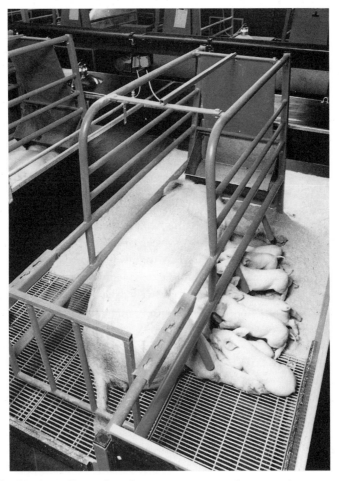

Fig. 6.1   Hygienically perfect farrowing accommodation with part-perforated floor.

Emphasis must also be placed on the importance of good feeding of the sow during pregnancy. Sufficient feed of good quality is essential for the production of piglets that can withstand the stress of the early days. Many problems have arisen because there has been a tendency to feed too lightly during pregnancy; sows become thin and unable to provide either sufficient nourishment for the development of the piglets or for the production of milk to feed them.

'Farrowing fever' (metritis, mastitis, agalactia syndrome or MMA)

A complex condition may occur in sows during the period of farrowing which seriously affects the viability of the piglets and the health of the sows. In this disease the sow runs an elevated temperature, usually about 40.5–42°C (105–107°F) and is quite ill, refusing food. Her skin is usually inflamed and the udder is often hard and tender. There will be little or no milk 'let-down' ('agalactia') and there is often inflammation of the uterus ('metritis'), which may be associated with retained afterbirths.

It is usually possible to cure the disease by immediate administration of broad-spectrum antibiotic injections such as amoxycillin, tetracyclines and potentiated sulphonamides and posterior pituitary hormone (oxytocin) to 'let down' the milk. It should be stressed that when 'farrowing fever' occurs it is a clear warning that certain changes in husbandry are required to try and prevent its recurrence. It is not usual for any specific infectious organism to be so involved that it can be said to be the certain cause. Essentially, the animal's resistance is in some way lowered so that such organisms that are normally present become invaders; these include bacteria such as *E. coli*, *Corynebacterium pyogenes*, staphylococci, streptococci and clostridia.

What are the factors which lower resistance? It is necessary to list a number, one or all of which may be involved. Some are easy to deal with, but others are more difficult: bad hygiene, overfeeding – giving rise to fat sows, inactivity during pregnancy and immaturity of the breeding herd may all play a part. Moving of pigs between herds can be an inciting cause, and assuredly the size and concentration of the unit will always tend to add to the problem. In many cases sows may be affected with some of the symptoms of the disease and then only relatively mildly. For example, it may be the agalactia alone or the mastitis that is clinically seen.

Farrowing fever is a syndrome often associated with undue pressure on space. Some farmers in desperation have put their sows to farrow in simple outdoor accommodation. This usually does the trick and yet no one is really any the wiser as to why. However, in diseases which are not caused by one factor but by several, the aim is to *reduce* the challenge as far as practicable as it is rarely possible to remove it completely under the restrictions of commercial farming.

It is essential with farrowing fever to ensure the quickest possible treatment of the sow so that she not only recovers but also provides the essential milk for the piglets. If she fails to make a quick response then it will be necessary either to foster her piglets or rear them artificially.

Diseases of young piglets

Escherichia coli infection

There are various ways in which this ubiquitous cause of trouble on the livestock farm can do damage. In the young pig, within the first few days of life, *E. coli* may be a cause of an acute septicaemic condition. Within only a few days of birth a number of pigs in the litter can become very ill with no particular symptoms except extreme illness leading to death.

Neonatal diarrhoea

Those pigs that are infected with *E. coli* but less seriously than those that succumb to the septicaemic form of the disease show a most serious, profuse watery diarrhoea. The piglets affected, whilst reasonably active and able to feed, nevertheless rapidly waste, have a staring coat and sunken eyes.

Milk scours and post-weaning diarrhoea

Another form of diarrhoea due to *E. coli* but occurring later is that known as 'milk scours'. A pale, greyish scour affects piglets in the period between 1 and 3 weeks of age and is very often associated with a change in the diet. Whilst under many circumstances the condition is quite transitory it may unfortunately become persistent and need treatment. Much the same can be said for post-weaning diarrhoea which affects pigs some 10 days after weaning. This is obviously induced by the changes in husbandry, housing and management, often exacerbated by bad hygiene and the mixing of too many piglets from too many different sources.

There are many strains of *E. coli* that cause these symptoms and almost certainly many of these strains will be living in perfect harmony within the intestines of the pig and will generally be present around the pigs' quarters. The *E. coli* appear to be able to multiply if there are certain stresses in the management and there are very many of these in the piglets' early. The first necessity in reducing the likelihood of infection with *E. coli* is to ensure that the piglets have a sufficient supply of colostrum. Thereafter changes should be as gradual or gentle as possible and this is often most difficult to achieve at or around the time of weaning. *Escherichia coli* often follows the occurrence of virus infections, many kinds of which are discussed throughout this chapter.

Treatment and prevention of *E. coli* and related infections

The treatment of *E. coli* infections is best achieved either by injections or medication incorporated in the feed or water. Many antibiotics can be used for this purpose, such as tetracyclines, amoxycillin, neomycin, Lincospectin, or potentiated sulphonamides. Neomycin, framomycin and others may be given orally.

The recovery of pigs suffering with *E. coli* diarrhoea will also be helped by administering fluids fortified with minerals, electrolytes and vitamins.

Prevention may be achieved by using certain broad-spectrum antibiotics or chemotherapeutics in the feed.

An alternative approach is to attempt to create an active or passive immunity by using serum or vaccine. The former course makes use of *E. coli* hyperimmune sera. In the case of vaccines, *E. coli* vaccine may be given to the sow during pregnancy or even to the piglets if there is adequate time before the problem would normally occur. In both cases at least two injections would be needed, some 14 days apart.

A more novel approach has been to incorporate mixed strains of killed *E. coli* in the sow's feed ('Intagen'). In many cases this method, as with the use of all vaccines, has been most successful but considerable variations are reported in its efficacy, due to the great variation in strains of bacteria. It must be emphasised again that the approach must always be to 'root out' the cause rather than 'add a vaccine' to the trouble.

Diseases of young and growing pigs

Transmissible gastroenteritis (TGE)

This is an alarming disease of pigs caused by a virus which is a comparative newcomer in the piglet field. When it strikes it tends to do so suddenly and will probably kill most of the piglets in a herd under 3 weeks of age. The symptom is a very severe diarrhoea which causes the piglets to die of dehydration. Some piglets vomit and all tend to have a very inflamed stomach and intestines, the sows may also be ill and have little milk. Pigs older than 3 weeks will also be affected to varying degrees and for a period will scour and make little progress. However, the symptoms in growing pigs may be so light as to go unnoticed.

The disease appears to have occurred with the growth of large herds. The virus sweeps across the whole herd like a bush fire and there is virtually nothing a farmer can do to protect his pigs. No vaccines are licensed for use in the UK, although they are available in some countries but are not of great value. However, after the disease has swept through the herd, the animals may be resistant to reinfection for some years. Even this statement, however, must be qualified since the nature of the virus seems to be constantly changing and variants may affect a herd soon after recovery from a previous attack, sometimes in a rather different way. For example, a variant may affect sows rather than piglets, the older the pig the worse being the effect.

In a large herd, virus infections like this may be rather slow to infect the herd and it is important to make every endeavour to get all the stock infected as quickly as possible to produce an immunity. This is most important with the young breeders, since they can then later produce viable litters. Ways of achieving this are to spread infected material, such as intestinal contents or even feeding homogenised piglets that have died from the disease; it seems a rather offensive method, and has the danger of spreading other infections, but it works. This procedure is, of course, in essence a crude way of live-vaccination and if it can be done sometime before the sow is due to farrow it should save the litter. A technique for the feed back routine is as follows. Twice a week remove some piglet faeces, mix with water in a bucket and give to sows and gilts due to farrow in the next 4–6 weeks. About 8–10 doses should be sufficient to stimulate the immunological system of the sow or gilt. Some attempts have also been made to give passive immunities by the use of serum from recovered pigs.

A good deal may be done to save piglets and lessen the effects in older pigs by feeding-up and nursing them by providing highly nutritious extra feed and additional comfort and warmth in the piggery.

Piglet anaemia

It can be said that every pig which is born in intensive housing requires some extra administration of iron to be sure that it does not become anaemic. It is interesting to study the reason for this. A piglet is born with limited reserves of iron in its liver, iron being an essential constituent of haemoglobin, the oxygen-carrying element in the red blood cells. There is also little iron in the sow's milk so the piglet will not get its requirement this way. Under natural conditions the piglet would be outside on pasture and would gain vital and sufficient quantities of iron from this source. However, no such source is available to the intensively housed pig and in any case modern pigs grow so quickly they more rapidly outstrip their limited reserve, so some supple-mentary source of assimilable iron must be given by solution, tablet, capsule or paste, or it is feasible to provide sods of grass or earth fortified with iron which the piglets can take in themselves. These are rather inexact ways of giving iron, so now it is almost always preferred to give the iron as an injection. It is usual to inject 200 mg of a soluble iron preparation when the piglet is not more than three days old and this is sufficient to carry it through to the time it is eating solid food, which should be liberally supplemented with iron.

Piglet anaemia may be recognised by pale, dull and hairy skins, scouring and exaggerated noisy heart beats – as the heart is overtaxed in an endeavour to increase the oxygen supply to the tissues. Diagnosis is confirmed by laboratory examination of the blood. Haemoglobin levels should be about 12 g/100 ml blood, but in anaemia the levels fall to 6 or less.

Bowel oedema

This is a rather curious disease of pigs which was once extremely common but now is more rarely seen, caused by certain strains of *E. coli* in the intestine. The condition almost invariably occurs about 10 days after weaning. The first indication of an outbreak is usually the appearance in a pen of weaners of one dead pig, often the biggest of the bunch. Close observation of others in the group may show they are suffering from various degrees of 'nervous trouble': staggering, incoordination, blindness, loss of balance and falling about when roused. As the disease progresses in these pigs they will lie on their side and paddle their legs and they then go into a coma and die within a day. In bowel oedema, such pigs usually show swollen (oedematous) eyelids, nose and ears and may have a moist squeal resembling a gurgle. A post mortem, if carried out speedily, shows oedema of the stomach and in the folds of the colon and in the larynx.

The occurrence of this disease seems to be associated with the stress of weaning, usually with the addition of *ad lib.* feeding when pigs may tend to eat too much, perhaps drink too little and become constipated, with their intestines engorged with high-quality diet. Under these circumstances it seems that certain strains of *E. coli* can multiply in the small intestine and produce toxins which do the damage.

Treatment is rarely successful but measures can be taken to prevent the spread of the disease, probably with success. All dry foods should be withdrawn and replaced with a limited wet diet. Pigs may be injected with broad-spectrum antibiotics, antihistamines and *E. coli* antiserum, and a saline purgative given. Consideration should be given to some change in the husbandry system that prevents pigs getting so much food at weaning; ideally a restricted wet feed would be given for a time.

Streptococcal infections

In recent years streptococcal infections of young piglets have become very common. The *Streptococcus suis* Type 1 infects the sow and she then transfers the infection to the piglets soon after birth. The organisms, after getting into the piglet, may cause a general infection (a septicaemia) which may cause immediate hyperacute infection and death or may be less acute and cause an endocarditis, meningitis and arthritis.

The disease usually occurs at abut 10 days of age. Affected pigs run a temperature, show painful arthritis, have muscular tremors, appear blind, and cannot coordinate their movements. Some die suddenly with heart inflammation. Typically, some 20–30% of a litter are affected.

Affected pigs may be treated successfully with injections of suitable antibiotics, such as penicillin or potentiated sulphonamides or broad-spectrum antibiotics. The disease tends to be a very tiresome herd problem and is often tackled by providing the sow with medicated feed. However, this is a very expensive way of dealing with the disease and good hygiene, 'isolation' farrowing and rearing are better.

A similar organism, *Streptococcus suis* Type 2, can also cause serious disease in older pigs. Here, what seems to happen is that young pigs, already carriers of the disease, are mixed with older pigs during the early fattening stages, say 8–12 weeks. The carriers infect the pigs they are mixed with and after a few days of incubation the affected pigs show a high temperature, nervous signs such as 'staggering', paralysis, arthritis and tetanic spasms: in other words, much the same signs as the younger pigs. Treatment is with penicillin or other antibiotics but the main requirement is to make sure that the cycle of infection is broken so infections do not take place.

Clostridial infections in pigs

Whilst the effects of clostridial infections on pigs are in no way comparable with those which affect sheep or even cattle, there are problems from time to time, particularly in outdoor-reared pigs on 'pig-sick' land.

For example, *Clostridium (perfringens)* can produce a fatal haemorrhagic enteritis in pigs up to about a week old. The disease has a very dramatic effect, with profuse dysentery, becoming dark from the profusion of blood within it. Usually affected pigs die very rapidly, although a few take a more chronic turn. Most die within 24 hours of the symptoms being noted. The litter affected should be treated with an antibiotic and those under risk of infection can be given lamb dysentery antiserum. A more permanent answer may be needed and the sows can be given a vaccine for the infection, this being administered twice during pregnancy.

Piglets are also infected with *Clostridium tetani* in the same way as lambs by penetration of the organism from dirty conditions, possibly through the navel or by the injury caused during castration or even by bad injection techniques, such as for anaemia. The signs are of stiffness and then tetanic spasms and death after the piglets have lain on their side with the limbs held out stiffly. The affected piglet usually dies, so the best course is to protect the other piglets and improve the hygiene of the pens and the management techniques.

Infections also occur with *Clostridium oedematiens*, which causes sudden death in breeding and fattening pigs, the latter usually in the later stages of growth. It usually affects pigs which are otherwise in very good health. The organism that causes the disease multiplies in the liver and produces the toxin that does the damage. It would seem that, with the liver active and vascular, the opportunity is provided for these organisms to invade the liver and multiply. If the problem threatens to be severe the antiserum may be used for immediate protection, and the vaccine can be used thereafter for long-term protection.

Greasy pig disease (exudative epidermitis; Marmite disease)

This is an acute skin inflammation of piglets with the production of excessive amounts of sebaceous secretion and exudation from the skin which does not cause irritation. It tends to be most common in hot weather. If it is severe, it leads to dehydration of the pig to such an extent that it dies. The actual cause of the disease is a bacterium, *Staphylococcus hyicus* but it is unlikely that it can produce this condition without prior injury in at least some of the piglets, for example from abrasions, from bad flooring or fittings and equipment, but it could also arise after a good deal of fighting and biting.

The condition usually occurs in piglets of about 2–8 weeks of age, and shows as a covering of the skin with an exudate of a greasy nature which mats the hair. The skin soon gets very dark, thickened and wrinkled and pigs lose weight and die. The number affected in a pig herd varies tremendously but normally only a modest number is affected. The best procedure after recognition of the condition is to inject a broad-spectrum antibiotic, such as ampicillin or lincomycin.

It is vital then to make sure that the cause is removed: in particular, the best procedure is to provide plenty of soft bedding. It is also believed that fortification of the feed with additional vitamins may assist in the ability of pigs to resist this condition.

Swine influenza

There have been a number of swine influenza virus strains found in pigs in the UK. The effect can be quite mild. An affected herd may show widespread fever, reduced appetite and a persistent cough for a few days, and then recover rapidly.

Unfortunately these uncomplicated cases are not the 'norm'. Very often secondary bacteria such as pasteurella invade the weakened respiratory tissues. Swine influenza is often associated with PRRS (p. 171) and together with secondaries leads to a serious and worrying drop in productivity, together with appalling food conversion efficiency.

So serious have been the combined effects of these pathogens that a number of farmers have reverted to keeping their stock under less-intensive methods in their determination to eliminate the effects of this range of infection.

Swine pox

This is a mild disease of world-wide incidence caused by a virus. It shows as red pimples (papules) over the abdomen which then become brown scabs and soon turn black; they will spread from the abdomen to other parts of the body and cause a slight general illness in the animal with a rise in temperature. The disease tends to occur in successive litters of young piglets but they normally recover quickly and are then immune to any further infection. The disease is mild so usually little is done to treat or prevent it but it is good to practise better disinfection procedures to try and eliminate it.

Atrophic rhinitis (AR)

Atrophic rhinitis (Fig. 6.2) is a respiratory disease caused principally by a bacterium, *Bordetella bronchiseptica*, and other organisms, notably a virus, the inclusion body rhinitis virus. Atrophic rhinitis primarily affects the membranes lining the delicate bones of the nose and leads to inflammation, nose bleeding, sneezing and eventually general degeneration of the bones of the snout. This does profound damage to the growth of the pig and it also makes the animal more susceptible to enzootic pneumonia and any infections of the respiratory tract.

This disease has become much more prevalent recently; it usually occurs in the early days of the pig's life and the increase in its occurrence has coincided with the advent of early weaning. This is not difficult to understand since pigs at this time are often kept in very close confinement in

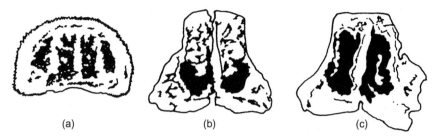

(a)   (b)   (c)

Fig. 6.2 Cross-section of pig's snout showing both normal and diseased turbinate bones after infection with atrophic rhinitis: (a) no atrophy of nasal turbinates; (b) typical atrophy of nasal turbinates; (c) severe atrophy of nasal turbinates.

kennels and other poorly ventilated accommodation at a time when their immunity to infection is at a minimum. Atrophic rhinitis may start a chain reaction with enzootic pneumonia in the fattening house as the final, economically disastrous outcome (see later in this chapter).

In order to prevent the condition a vaccine may be used, or continuous preventive medication may be instituted with a suitable antibiotic, such as tylosin, or a chemotherapeutic drug such as a sulphonamide. It is essentially better to improve the environment and management than to rely on measures of vaccination and medication. The procedures listed under enzootic pneumonia are equally applicable to AR.

Diseases largely of fatteners

Salmonellosis

All forms of salmonellosis can occur in pigs but there are a number of serious ones which are a matter of great practical concern, especially because of the dangers of contamination of the human food supply. *Salmonella typhimurium* is a virulent salmonella to all livestock and man and is common enough to warrant special care. On the other hand, the purely pig pathogen *S. cholerae suis*, which was once a frequent problem, is now quite rare. There are a great number of salmonellae of 'exotic' type which come from the pigs' feed but these do not tend to cause serious difficulties for long.

Symptoms vary tremendously, depending on the type and virulence of the salmonellae. All ages can be affected but the worst outbreaks seem to be after weaning, in large groups of 'stores'. Salmonellosis often shows itself in the septicaemic form, causing sudden death or acute fever with blue (cyanotic) discolouration of the ears and limbs. Another form of disease shows itself as acute diarrhoea, also with a fever, but these are not all the signs.

Pneumonia may occur with abnormal breathing and also nervous abnormalities, such as incoordination and paralysis. Also, the skin is often affected and parts may even 'slough-off' later in the disease. In more chronic forms, pigs may be in a state of almost perpetual diarrhoea, eating yet still wasting. A very high proportion of a group or pen may be affected so the economic effects are very serious.

Diagnosis by an expert is essential and the laboratory can arrange for 'typing' of the organism; this is often important if the cause of the infection is to be traced.

In order to deal with the disease, a number of measures are advised; it is such a serious infection that it is vital that *all* of these are taken. First, it is necessary to treat infected animals. This will require drugs or antibiotics with known activity against salmonella, such as enrofloxacins, amoxycillin, potentiated sulphonamides and streptomycin, administered by injection or in the water or feed, depending on the product. The best technique is to give an initial injection to each pig individually and then follow this with medication in the drinking water.

The only form of salmonella that can be prevented by vaccination is *S. cholerae suis*. A general preventive measure is to isolate the pigs from their own excreta, so far as possible, and also to prevent cross-infection of excreta from pen to pen. Feedstuffs may be monitored by a laboratory for salmonella, but the pelleting process itself goes some way to limit the possibilities of infection. Feed may also be specially heat-treated or may have the addition of special products to kill any salmonella organism that may be present. If rats or other rodents could be the cause of disease, a 'blitz' on their presence is called for. It may also be necessary to carry out more careful isolation of pigs that are possibly carriers. It would certainly be advisable to take the greatest care in disinfecting all contaminated areas and to institute a more thorough process than hitherto. With salmonella it may also be necessary to consider staff testing because on several occasions in the author's experience it has been the stockmen who have been the carriers of the infection. Salmonellosis is a notifiable disease under the Zoonoses Order in the UK (see also Chapter 3).

Enzootic pneumonia

One of the most serious scourges and causes of economic loss on the pig farm is the disease of pneumonia caused by a species of mycoplasma: *M. hyopneumoniae*. Although this is recognised as the principal cause of the disease, other organisms are commonly secondary invaders, including other types of mycoplasma and bacteria, such as *Pasteurella multicoida* and *Bordetella bronchiseptica.* The lesions of enzootic pneumonia tend to be in the anterior lobes of the lungs, which become consolidated (solid) and grey in colour. The disease is readily recognised by the constant harsh coughing of pigs in the fattening house.

Treatment with medicines should be instituted in pigs showing serious clinical signs. Broad-spectrum antibiotics such as tetracyclines or amoxycillin may be injected but may not have a permanent beneficial effect as no immunity follows an attack. A vaccine is now available, Suvaxyn, which is very effective in reducing the effects of the disease.

Whilst the final effects of this disease may be to kill a proportion of pigs, chiefly in the fattening house, its most serious effect is to lower the growth rate and food conversion efficiency of nearly all the animals in the building. In addition, badly infected stock may require constant treatment, so that considerable medication costs have to be faced.

There is no doubt that it is ideal to have stock that are entirely free of the infectious agent that is primarily responsible, such animals are available and a very small proportion of herds maintain this status. In total, however, they are a minute percentage of the national herd and many herds that were free have broken down. Thus it is pertinent to consider how one deals with this problem environmentally in an infected herd, this is the surest way of minimising the effects.

The first essential is to start, if possible, in a building which is free of all stock and then 'batch' the groups of fatteners through the building. If this is impossible, the next best thing is to subdivide the building so that each section can be dealt with in this way.

There is, in any case, considerable virtue in limiting the number of pigs in one air space since it makes a build-up of infection less likely and enables the environment to be more satisfactorily maintained. Ventilation is easier, draughts are less likely and heat is better conserved.

Virtually all those factors which enable good ventilation will assist in reducing the effects of enzootic pneumonia. Ventilation must never be sacrificed in order to maintain temperature. Air flow must be arranged so that it takes fresh air to the pigs before it moves over dung or slurry. All gases that emanate from the slurry channels must be taken immediately out of the house. Condensation must be prevented and this is often only achieved by good thermal insulation of the surfaces. Cold and damp are the most lethal combinations; insulation assists the maintenance of good temperature.

It is also important to stock the house as lightly as is compatible with good economy and also subdivide the unit into as small pen sizes as possible; this will help to ensure a fairly uniform distribution of the pigs through the house and prevent overcrowding in limited areas.

Swine dysentery ('bloody scours')

This is an infection which has probably affected pigs at least in a limited way for as long as pigs have been raised intensively but which has only recently come into major prominence. It is a disease largely of fattening pigs and the infection causes inflammation of the intestines, leading to dysentery (diarrhoea together with some bloody effusions) and general debilitation. It is highly contagious, being spread via contact with infected faeces, and it is of course readily understandable that it has become a more common disease in recent years, since modern intensification has brought much larger numbers of pigs together and there is a greater opportunity for the spread of infection. Furthermore, certain changes in husbandry practices have apparently contributed to the increased incidence of infection. The absence of bedding to absorb or dilute the pigs' faeces and urine has made for close contact between the pig and its excreta. The use of slatted floors of imperfect design often leads to a build-up of faeces in dark and ill-ventilated corners which may hardly ever be cleaned out. Another major contributory cause has been the practice of feeding on the floor. This is a good procedure if the floor conditions are good and the pigs are eating off a clean surface; if, however, the floor is contaminated with excreta and the food is thrown on top of this, it needs little imagination to realise the easy way in which infection can be spread and it becomes an appalling arrangement.

The main causal organism involved in swine dysentery is a bacterium, *Treponema hyodysenteriae*, although it is not the only one involved and others such as *Vibrio coli, E. coli* and salmonellae of various species may be present as secondaries.

Early recognition of the disease is important. Affected pigs swish their tails; at the same time there may be diarrhoea and if this is examined more closely there will be streaks of blood, mucus and some pieces of the lining of the intestine which have come away (necrotic material). The faeces have a characteristically unpleasant smell. As the condition progresses the affected pigs gradually waste and may show a capricious appetite but they still drink freely. Swine dysentery primarily affects the large intestine which, on post mortem, shows degenerative changes.

Treatment

A number of useful medicines may be given via the food or water, the latter route being preferable since sick pigs will drink but may not eat. The range of medicines used includes tylosin, erythromycin, spiramycin, sulpha drugs, lincomycin, Lincospectin and tiamulin.

It can be seen that the range of medicines is very extensive but complete reliance should not be put on medication. Systems of husbandry which tend to produce swine dysentery should be modified to reduce the danger, i.e. by disinfection, isolation and improvement in dung disposal arrangements.

The intestinal haemorrhage syndrome ('bloody gut')

The condition, often known as 'bloody gut', affects fatteners in the later stages of their growth. After a short period of depression, with an appearance of paleness and an enlarged abdomen, they die rapidly. Post-mortem examination shows the small intestine full of blood-stained fluid and gas in the large intestine, there may also be a twisting of the gut.

The condition is more common in whey-fed pigs, but not exclusively so, and its cause remains a mystery.

Mulberry heart disease

This is a rather curious disease, mostly of fatteners over the weight of about 45 kg (100 lb). The symptoms are either sudden death or the pigs become depressed and weak and collapse and die within about 24 hours of the onset of the disease. Few pigs ever recover. On post-mortem examination the signs are of an enlarged and mottled liver and the surface of the heart is streaked with haemorrhages running longitudinally and also occurring in the endocardium. The cause is not really known but there is a suggestion that a deficiency of Vitamin E or selenium may be involved. There is little evidence that treatment does much good but the use of multi-vitamin injections and broad-spectrum antibiotics may be of some benefit. The range of medicines is very extensive but, again, there should not be too much dependence on these.

Porcine reproductive and respiratory system (PRRS)

This is a new disease of pigs that only appeared in Europe in late 1990, and in the UK the first case was reported in May 1991, where it is still often referred to as blue-ear pig disease. The disease was first described in the USA in 1987 and is now probably world-wide. It is a good example of the 'viral strike': a condition caused by several different strains of an arterivirus (or the Lelystad virus) causing a variety of symptoms. It is an extremely contagious condition, capable of spreading at least 20 km by the windborne route. Attempts to limit its spread in the UK and elsewhere have proved fruitless.

The signs of the disease are very variable. In sows the signs are depression, inappetence, breeding abnormalities of every sort, abortions at any stage, premature farrowing, agalactia, respiratory symptoms such as coughing and distress, and finally cyanosis of the ears (hence 'blue-ear') and vulva, snout and teats. The variation in cyanosis is enormous, sometimes being very transitory but in other cases leading to necrosis. In boars similar symptoms may be seen as in the sow but the quality of the semen is likely to be reduced for some weeks.

In piglets the signs of PRRS include marked neonatal diarrhoea which responds poorly to treatment, increased overall mortality, reduced birth-weight, an increased number of stillborn mummified piglets, respiratory distress and all manner of secondary infections causing lameness and greasy skins.

In infected growers and finishing pigs there may be no signs of illness, alternatively, very serious pneumonia problems may develop.

To back up the symptoms, positive diagnosis of the condition can be made by serology. Treatment can only attempt to alleviate secondary bacterial infection with such measures as broad-spectrum antibiotics, electrolytes, vitamins and minerals and generally improved nutrition.

As the disease has spread the symptoms have become less pronounced and indeed it is no longer the scourge it was. The pig population now 'carries' the milder strains of the virus which in effect act similarly to a vaccine.

Disease of pigs largely without age incidence

Swine erysipelas ('the diamonds')

A bacterium known as *Erysipelothrix insidiosa* or *E. rhusiopathiae* is one of the most common causes of disease in pigs. Most pigs are under risk of this disease because the organism can live in and around piggeries and 'pig-sick' land for very many years in the sporulated form. It is found mostly in breeding pigs but it can occur in pigs of all ages. It manifests itself in a number of entirely different ways. In the peracute form of the disease there may be hardly any signs at all, and the pig may be found dead after a very brief period of severe illness. In the acute form the pig is also ill, has a high temperature, the skin is inflamed and it will not eat. Then there is a sub-acute form which is the more typical disease, showing characteristic dis-coloration of the skin with raised purplish areas (said to be roughly diamond-shaped) throughout the back and on the flanks and belly. Finally, there are two chronic forms of the disease; in one the joints are affected, which causes the pig severe lameness, whilst in the other the organism causes erosion of the valves of the heart, leading to cauliflower-like growths, so that the pig will often show signs of heart dysfunction or even heart failure and death. If pregnant sows are affected they will almost certainly abort. A feature of swine erysipelas is that it tends to affect pigs during hot and muggy weather conditions; for some reason such stressful conditions favour the multiplication of the organisms and the infection of the pigs. Indeed, any stressful conditions will increase the risk.

It is clear that there are very serious effects on pigs of all ages and a programme of protection is necessary on farms where the trouble commonly occurs.

Good vaccines which will protect a pig for about 1 year are available. Affected pigs can be treated with the hyperimmune antiserium or an antibiotic, penicillin being totally effective. In-contact pigs may be protected with the antiserum or penicillin. When the condition arises in a herd it is usual for it to have quite a limited effect in the first instance but to gradually rise in severity as the disease progresses; thus it is vital to deal with the condition at once. Vaccines protect for up to a year and it is usually only the breeder pigs which require protection on an annual basis before the summer weather.

Heat stroke

Many pigs are lost from this cause, certainly many more than suspected. It happens under almost any circumstances when pigs are kept in a temperature of above about 32°C if the air circulation is bad and the pig has no way of cooling itself by 'wallowing'. The pig has virtually no sweat glands so it can keep cool only by increasing respirations (panting) or by wallowing in water and allowing evaporation of the water to cool it. Wallowing is virtually never possible under intensive conditions of husbandry and indeed when it does happen it is usually done in the dunging passage in a mixture of the pigs' urine, faeces and drinking water; such a procedure makes attempts at disease control a potential disaster!

If pigs are found suffering with heat stroke, immediate cooling with cold water as rapidly as possible, with good air movement created in the surroundings, is an absolute necessity and is often much more successful than appears likely. It is also useful to spray water in the building as an emergency measure using, if possible, a horticultural type of spray applicator. It is also a good policy to drip water over the roof or walls of the building and in mechanically ventilated buildings it is useful to trickle water over the inlets. Some mention should be made of the so-called 'sweat box' system of rearing fatteners in accommodation that is kept at a deliberately high temperature and humidity. Apart from the fact that this contravenes the pigs' welfare code in the UK, it is noteworthy that it may also cause heat stroke because the margin between a high figure which is safe (about 28°C) and one which is lethal (say 32°C) is a rather thin one. Also, whilst the system appears to be tolerated by pigs if the humidity is high and the floor wet, no such tolerance is apparent if the air becomes dry and the pigs cannot wallow to keep cool.

Swine fever (hog cholera)

This is a virus disease of pigs formerly of worldwide incidence. It is still probably the most serious of all pig diseases, although it has now been eliminated from many countries, including the UK. Swine fever affects pigs of all ages. When it first affects a herd it is more likely to occur in the acute form, with the pigs showing a very high temperature, great depression and discoloration of the skin. Less acute cases may occur at the same time; in these cases pigs have a fever and usually diarrhoea of a particularly foetid type. Pigs also have a depraved appetite and thirst. This highly contagious disease will also manifest itself in other forms – the pneumonic form characterised by respiratory illness; the skin form showing itself as ulcers and plaques on the skin; and the nervous type leading to incoordination, paralysis and death. The most likely outcome of infection of a herd with swine fever, if it is allowed to run on, is to find a considerable proportion of the pigs with a chronic scour which hardly responds at all to any treatment, so that the pigs continue to lose weight.

In this country swine fever has been controlled for many years by a slaughter policy. Elsewhere it may be controlled by vaccination, but there is little doubt that the slaughter policy, if it can be achieved to eliminate the disease altogether, is by far the most economic method.

There is also a highly virulent disease, with symptoms rather like swine fever, known as African swine fever. However, although the symptoms are much the same, it is caused by a completely different virus. It has a devastating effect and may kill 90% of the pigs in a herd or even more. Until recent years it occurred only in Africa but recently it has occurred in parts of southern Europe; it has been eliminated from France and Italy. Should it occur in the UK it would undoubtedly be dealt with by a slaughter policy. There are import restrictions on pigs or pig products from areas where African swine fever is present.

Aujeszky's disease

This is currently of much concern as a disease in Europe, although not in the UK, and in many other parts of the world. It is an infection caused by a herpes virus which leads to nervous and respiratory symptoms with a fever. Death often occurs in young pigs. In adults there may be few, if any, signs but sows will often abort or their litters will be stillborn, if they are affected. It is a notifiable disease in the UK and the national herd is currently free of the disease.

Infection with Aujeszky's disease virus occurs in the epithelium of the upper respiratory tract and multiplication of the virus here is followed by its spread into the nervous system, but some strains of the virus also produce pneumonia. The virus also invades the uterus to cause abortions, stillbirths, mummification and foetal resorption.

The mortality in the piglet affected up to about 4 weeks of age may reach 100% but in the older piglet it is likely to be below 50%, up to about 8 weeks. Above this age range the effects are much more slight or animals may even be symptomless carriers.

In young animals clinical signs which may be seen are vomiting, diarrhoea, trembling, incoordination, muscular spasms and convulsions. A certain diagnosis can only be made by serological tests in the laboratory. The disease is very widespread in some countries and 'carrier' pigs easily spread this very contagious disease. It is much more likely to be of economic importance with big herds of 250 sows and above.

There is no treatment of any use. Prevention is achieved by the use of live attenuated and dead virus vaccines in many countries, including the USA, Europe and Northern Ireland, but no licence has yet been given for its use in the UK. It is possible to test, remove reactors and possibly eliminate the disease, but there is no agreement whether to use vaccine as the best control method, or whether to test and slaughter.

Leptospirosis

Two species of the bacteria *Leptospira* (*L. canicola* and *L. icterohaemorrhagiae*) affect pigs. The disease they cause varies in its symptoms depending upon the acuteness of the infection. In young pigs there is usually some fever (temperature about 40°C: 106°F) and diarrhoea and jaundice (yellowing). In breeding pigs the disease will often cause abortion and stillbirths, together with sickness in the sow. Post-mortem lesions tend to be largely confined to the kidney, a greyish-white lesion appearing in the cortex of the kidney. Diagnosis is confirmed by isolation of the organism from the pig, usually via the urine. Many pigs may be symptomless carriers of the disease.

The disease is picked up from carrier pigs or from rodents which frequently carry the disease under rather unsanitary conditions. In overtly sick animals, antibiotics may be used successfully. Rodents should be eliminated as far as possible and disinfection programmes improved.

Anthrax

The bacterium *Bacillus anthracis*, which is so serious a cause of sudden death in cattle, also infects pigs but causes different symptoms. Infection usually comes into the herd via infected animal products in the feed, the organism entering through the throat glands. A common symptom is oedema and swelling of the neck region, with difficult breathing and a very high temperature: up to 40.5°C (107°F). In younger pigs the disease may just cause sudden death without any symptoms showing at all.

Penicillin is the most effective treatment and this or a specific antiserum can be used to treat and prevent infection.

Anthrax is a notifiable disease and is potentially very dangerous to man. Thus the diagnosis should be undertaken by a veterinarian if the disease is suspected and thereafter, if confirmed, appropriate official action will be advised and taken (see also the section on anthrax in Chapter 5).

Tuberculosis in pigs

Three forms of tuberculosis – bovine, avian and human – can infect the pig. Because of the much reduced incidence of tuberculosis in cattle and man, there is now very little in pigs but it does still exist as a clinical entity. Of the cases that occur, most are of the avian type, doubtless infected by wild birds since tuberculosis is virtually non-existent in domestic fowl.

The symptoms are rather non-specific and would rarely be suspected by the pigman. Loss of weight, coughing and discharge from the nose will hardly lead to suspicion, so it is unusual for the disease to be recognised before it is detected in the slaughterhouse by the presence of swollen and infected lymph nodes in the throat, chest and abdomen. If samples are taken the disease can then be diagnosed positively.

Treatment is rarely called for but careful consideration should be given to isolating stock from sources of infection and improving the hygiene of the premises. The organisms that cause tuberculosis in all species are very persistent and resist destruction by most means; it is therefore very important to take such measures that eliminate them. It is also pertinent to stress the risk to the human population and whilst it is not a highly contagious agent of disease, it could represent a very undesirable challenge to man if the infection became widespread in a pig herd.

Mycotoxicosis

Pigs, like all farm animals, can be affected by poisonous substances – mycotoxins – which can be formed in the feed as a result of the growth of fungi. Effects vary, depending on the fungi involved and the toxins produced, from abortion and stillbirths to a condition where there is no more than reduced growth, weight loss, jaundice and undersized pigs. The former is often caused by fusarium poisoning, the latter by *Aspergillus flavus* (aflactoxicosis). This organism is a common contaminant of groundnuts which, because of this problem, are now rarely used for feeding to livestock. Ergot poisoning also occurs occasionally when grain contaminated with ergot, another fungus, is fed to pigs; it causes agalactia and the birth of small or weak piglets.

There is no effective treatment for poisoning by mycotoxins. Diagnosis is sometimes quite difficult and depends on specialist laboratory examination. Obviously prevention lies in removing the contaminated feedstuffs from the animals. A number of chemicals that can be placed in the food to inhibit fungal growth are now available.

The farmer can do little or nothing about cereals imported on to his premises but it is known that one of the problems that can arise is due to the growth of fungus in the bulk bin and these should receive periodical cleanouts and then treatment with antifungal agents to take care of the next batch of bulk food.

Gas poisoning

There have been many cases of serious losses in pigs, and even danger to the pigman, from toxic gases. Whilst these mostly arise from the slurry under slatted floor channels, sometimes carbon monoxide can be generated from incomplete or inefficient combustion of gas in gas heaters. The result may be death in the young piglet or the sow may abort her litter (see Chapter 1).

Foot-and-mouth disease

This disease, notifiable in the Uk, and its importance is fully discussed in Chapter 5. Three special points may, however, be made with regard to the disease in pigs. Firstly, symptoms of lameness are more often the first signs of illness, whereas in cattle the vesicles on the mouth are usually the first symptoms. Secondly, primary outbreaks can well occur in pigs fed infected meat products that have been improperly sterilised. The final point is that the symptoms are largely indistinguishable from swine vesicular disease, which is also a viral and notifiable disease but which only affects pigs.

Swine vesicular disease (SVD)

This is another condition caused by an enterovirus and was first recognised in the UK in 1972. Since then it has been a sporadically occurring infection. Clinical signs are similar to foot-and-mouth disease, including lameness due to inflammation and vesicles developing on the foot and also on the mouth, tongue and areas of the skin over the legs. Affected pigs may also show some nervous symptoms.

SVD is a highly contagious infection but the effect on pigs is relatively mild. Nevertheless, in view of its similarity to foot-and-mouth disease, a positive diagnosis being possible only at a specialist laboratory, the two diseases are dealt with in exactly the same way by slaughtering all infected and in-contact stock.

Rabies

The virus that affects all mammals (see Chapter 5) may very rarely affect pigs in rabies-infected areas. It will cause much the same symptoms of incoordination, salivation, muscular spasms, paralysis and death within about 3–4 days from the onset of the symptoms.

Important virus infections affecting pigs of various ages

Pig enterovirus infections, including 'SMEDI'

A popular discussion point of pig farmers is the condition known as 'SMEDI' – stillbirth, mummification, embryonic death and infertility. The condition is caused by various enteroviruses. Suspicion of this condition will be aroused when the various symptoms listed occur, and it is important for the farmer to obtain a specialist diagnosis before appropriate control measures can be taken, which will have to be along the same lines as the parvovirus problem (see later in this chapter). The process of 'feeding-back' infected material to act as a vaccine, however, is very risky because it may spread diseases other than the particular infection which is causing concern; a laboratory diagnosis can help to reduce this risk by establishing that the pigs are not otherwise diseased.

Pig enteroviruses may also be associated with nervous symptoms not dissimilar to poliomyelitis in man. Affected animals run a high temperature and show incoordination, followed by stiffness, tremors and convulsions and most pigs then die within a week of infection. This condition will occur in all pigs in herds which are non-immune and where the disease is enzootic; it may also occur in a mild, less serious form in which the pigs have fever and show some incoordination which is often followed by recovery, although some become paralysed and have to be culled.

The acute form of this disease, known as Teschen disease, is probably not present in the UK but it is a notifiable disease and would be dealt with by a slaughter policy to attempt to eradicate it. The mild form, known as Talfan disease, is certainly present in the UK but no special control policies are instituted and reliance is placed on the pigs developing a natural immunity, as with many other virus diseases of rather mild and uncertain symptoms. Vaccines are available although none are licensed in the UK (see earlier in this chapter under TGE).

Rotavirus infection

Rotavirus infection causes very severe scouring in piglets which can lead to quite a heavy mortality. The symptoms are anorexia, vomiting and diarrhoea which is yellow or dark grey in colour and very profuse. The diarrhoea causes rapid dehydration which can kill, otherwise the pigs can recover in about a week to 10 days.

These clinical signs are very similar to other conditions of young pigs causing profuse diarrhoea, such as TGE and *E. coli* infection and only a laboratory diagnosis to identify the virus will confirm the cause. There are no specific control measures and reliance will have to be placed on endeavouring to provide good nursing for the affected piglets, with generalised treatment to deal with secondaries.

Vomiting and wasting disease

This is a disease of the newborn pig caused by a coronavirus similar to the TGE virus. Affected pigs vomit, huddle together with general illness, are depressed, run a high temperature and show little interest in suckling. Only a proportion of piglets in a litter are affected and only a proportion of all litters may be affected at all.

Parvovirus infection

Parvovirus infection of pigs is a cause of infertility, stillbirths, small litters and mummification. It is a relatively new condition that has been recognised in a number of large units. It tends to be most commonly seen in young gilts or newly introduced pigs which have no resistance to the 'local' infection but it may also infect boars which then act as spreaders of infection. It appears to be far more of a problem in those housing systems where the sows are kept as individuals (as in tethering or sow stalls) and where the lack of contact fails to produce a passing infection and then resistance. In this type of condition there is no treatment that is of any real use. No licensed vaccines have been produced in the UK but none are really recommended elsewhere. One procedure is to 'infect' a young gilt before service and the most effective way is to 'feed' homogenised placenta from known infected cases.

Epidemic diarrhoea

This is a very contagious disease of pigs caused by a virus which produces a profuse diarrhoea, vomiting, wasting and inappetence. The disease is similar to TGE but largely affects older pigs; younger pigs are affected either very much less or not at all. The effects of the virus vary a great deal but generally they are serious and many piglets die due to the inability of the sow to suckle them. Also, quite a number of sows will show such wasting that they may never breed again and have to be culled. There is little that can be done. It is suggested that all sows within about 2 weeks of farrowing are isolated. On the other hand, those that are in earlier stages of pregnancy than this should be deliberately infected with the virus by mixing with carriers or using dung or infected material. It is difficult to quickly achieve total infection and consequent immunity in the herd and the crude methods that seem necessary to accelerate the build-up of immunity may be harmful in other respects if other infections are spread.

Epidemic diarrhoea is another infection of a viral origin which seems to pass by smaller herds yet have a devastating effect on the larger ones; this is a further argument for establishing and maintaining breeding herds of a modest size. One of the greatest difficulties is to obtain a reasonably speedy total infection and consequent immunity in the herd but the crude measures that seem necessary to accelerate the build-up of immunity may be quite harmful in other respects by spreading other infections. This is a further argument in favour of establishing and maintaining breeding herds of a modest size where such problems do not occur or, if they do, have minimal effects.

General control measures for virus infections when no vaccines are available

The upsurge in the number of virus infections in pig herds in recent years is worrying and provides us with lessons of great importance. These infections appear to be very similar to those conditions that have affected poultry but the pig industry is much more vulnerable; it tends to be more careless about hygiene, has no general policy of depopulation of sites and generally moves pigs around during their lifetime much more than is the case with poultry.

To minimise the effects of disease, the following preventive measures should be considered:

(1) Introduce a minimum of new stock from outside the unit
(2) Depopulate the housing of young pigs as frequently as possible
(3) Keep adult breeders closely but cleanly housed
(4) Do not use sow stalls or tethers but use kennels or yards which group the gilts, sows and boars. Sow stalls and tethers will in any case be illegal in the UK on welfare grounds
(5) Limit the size of each self-contained unit to a minimum. This will quickly reduce the effects of any virulent viruses in the area
(6) Practise careful isolation of the site in terms of feed deliveries, visitors, collecting lorries for fat pigs and any other potential danger

External parasites

Pigs may be quite badly infected with lice (*Haematopinus suis*), the mange mite (*Sarcoptes scabei* var. suis) and the stable fly (*Stomoxys calcitrans*).

Lice

Lice tend to be most common in the folds of the skin of the neck, around the base of the ears, on the insides of the legs and on the flanks. The louse is quite large – about 0.5 mm long – and can be seen moving amongst the hairs on the pig's skin. The constant irritation causes the pig to rub and scratch and this reduces growth and food conversion efficiency. Also, the lice may be vectors of other disease agents.

Knowledge of the life-cycle of the pig louse assists in effecting control measures. The lice lay their eggs on the bristles and can be seen as a yellow crust. The eggs hatch into a nympth in 10–20 days, then after two further nymphal stages the life-cycle is completed in about 30 days. The lice can only live away from the host for 2–3 days and the pig is the only host.

Because lice cause considerable economic loss it is unwise to tolerate an infection. The best way of dealing with the problem is to treat all sows just before they enter farrowing accommodation. Suitable preparations are based on deltamethrin.

Mange

Mange is an infinitely more worrying problem than lice. The parasite which is most common in the pig (*Sarcoptes scabei* var. suis) burrows in the skin and lives in so-called 'galleries'. The mange parasites are about 0.5 mm long and lay their eggs in the galleries and develop through larval and two nymphal stages to adults within a period of about 15 days. Whilst the parasites can multiply only on the pig, the mites can survive up to 2–3 weeks in piggeries.

The burrowing and feeding of the mites cause considerable damage to the skin and intense irritation. Fluid exudate oozes from the lesions and dries and causes crusts on the skin. The skin becomes grossly thickened and keratinised and may also become infected with bacteria. In the final stages of the disease the skin looks more like that of an elephant than a pig.

The disease has important economic considerations and must be eliminated if pigs are to thrive. Suitable preparations for treatment are phosmet, diazinon, and bromocyclen. Two applications at intervals of 10 days may be fully successful. If such pigs are then put into completely clean accommodation it is feasible to eliminate the disease or at least reduce it to a very low level.

Internal parasites

Not many years ago the various internal parasites of pigs constituted a major problem in pig husbandry but that situation is largely over. For one thing, the adoption of more intensive systems has tended to eliminate the secondary hosts which have an essential role in the life-cycles of some parasites. And for another, modern anthelmintics are so effective that treatment and prevention enable the problem to be readily resolved. The main concern to the pig farmer is subclinical infection which may go undetected while in reality doing great harm. It is also pertinent to observe that as there is some movement back to less-intensive methods, with pigs grazing outdoors, there may be a resurgence of internal parasites.

Ascariasis

Ascaris lumbricoides is the common large roundworm that lives in the small intestine. Some can achieve a length of up to 450 mm. Infection can be so bad that the intestines are literally blocked with large numbers of these worms. In any event, the presence of worms invariably leads to some deterioration in the food conversion and growth efficiency. However, these are not really the worst effects of this particular infection. The life-cycle is direct – no intermediate host is involved – and after the eggs are laid and ingested by pigs kept under unhygienic conditions, the eggs hatch out and the larvae, in their development to the adult stage, which is always in the intestine, actually pass through the lungs and liver. Coughing and pneumonia result from the migration of the larvae in the lungs, and the damage by the larvae almost certainly allows bacteria to invade and cause secondary symptoms. The effect on the liver appears to be slight because the pigs usually show no symptoms. The tracking of the larvae through the liver does do some damage, however, leaving small white areas known as 'milk spots', so it is possible to tell at post mortem, or at the slaughterhouse, that the worms have caused damage. These signs provide a good warning to the pig farmer. In addition the livers may be condemned as being unfit for human consumption.

Control can be relatively easy as the life-cycle is a direct one. If pigs can be prevented from reinfesting themselves by ingesting anything which is contaminated with their faeces the life-cycle can be broken. One must beware of dirty pens, floor feeding, dirty troughs, contaminated drinking water or 'pig-sick' land. Good disinfectants will kill the eggs or larvae. Treatment of the pigs with anthelmintics will eliminate the worms. The condition should not be tolerated and a campaign to eliminate the worms will have beneficial effects, not only by eliminating these worms but also other susceptible types.

Other intestinal worms of pigs occur in various parts of the intestine, including the two stomach worms *Ostertagia* and *Hyostrongylus rubidus*. These are small reddish worms about 10 mm long which infect the stomach lining, chiefly affecting and causing damage to sows. Clinically infection causes weight loss and anaemia in sows, mainly after weaning. Infection is most likely to arise when the sows are put on to pasture after weaning for service with the boar. Also common in breeding pigs is the worm *Oesophagostomum*. This is a worm of about 15 mm in length which is found in the caecum and colon. Again, it has a direct life-cycle and it causes diarrhoea and weight loss; it is associated with dirty paddocks.

Finally, there is a lungworm of importance known as *Metastrongylus*. The adult worm lives in the bronchioles of the lungs. In this case the life-cycle is indirect, infection being caused by ingestion of the earthworm which is the intermediate host of the *Metastrongylus* larvae. The lungworms undoubtedly cause damage to the lungs and pneumonia, but it is chiefly in younger pigs that the symptoms are serious. Older pigs are not usually adversely affected but do remain as carriers of the infection.

Control of the endoparasites

Symptoms such as those described give an indication of the identity of the infection but it is important that an expert parasitologist conducts a proper laboratory examination to give an accurate diagnosis. Usually treatments are carried out by in-feed medication of suitable products, such as fenbendazole, tetramisole, thiabendazole, piperazines and dichlorvos.

Regular programmes should be instituted where problems exist, according to the direction of the manufacturers.

Deficiency diseases

Because pigs are usually fed efficiently calculated and mixed rations, deficiencies of vitamins, minerals and other food substances are uncommon. Nevertheless, one still has to be closely aware of the possibility that deficiencies may arise. Sometimes the essential ingredients are missing due to error, but more often deficiencies arise because the element is not available. For example, *Parakeratosis* is an absolute or conditioned efficiency of zinc which causes poor growth and hyperkeratosis, the latter being a proliferation of the epidermis causing scaly, crusty skin, especially on the abdomen and legs. It is readily dealt with by ensuring a level of 100 ppm of zinc in the ration.

As a second example, the B group vitamin biotin may need supplementing. Deficiencies cause scaly skin and lameness due to cracking of the horn of the feet (Fig. 6.3). Levels up to 220 micrograms per kilogram are required in the diet. High-energy feeds with a cereal basis of only wheat and barley, but no maize, appear to be the cause of the trouble.

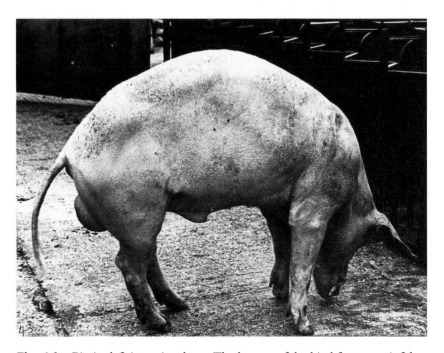

Fig. 6.3 Biotin deficiency in a boar. The hooves of the hind feet are painful as a result of the damaged soft horn. The pig stands uncomfortably to relieve the weight on them with a typical hunched-back stance. Poor, dirty skin is also seen.

Foot and leg lesions in pigs

Warning must be given that many pigs, especially young piglets, suffer damage to their feet and legs due to unsatisfactory flooring. Rough concrete floors cause sore feet and serious abrasions on the knees and legs. In addition, slatted or slotted flooring can cause even more serious and penetrating damage due to poor design and sharp edges. Parts of the foot can literally be torn off. Apart from the immediate damage and pain caused in all these cases, secondary infection can readily set in to cause highly destructive damage to the tissue.

Lameness in older pigs may be caused by foot rot, an infection affecting the claws of the feet and causing penetrating damage and erosion. The primary cause is probably an injury, then secondary infection with bacteria, such as *Fusiformis necrophorus* (see Chapters 5 and 7) follows. The lameness created can be serious and the lesions so penetrating that no treatment can arrest the process of tissue destruction. Lameness is also caused by abnormal or excess growth of the claws. All these conditions may be caused by keeping pigs on soft and wet flooring, with insufficient exercise. Good, clean straw bedding can be a perfect surface but if it is not renewed frequently the consequences can be disastrous.

It is estimated that foot and leg lesions together are responsible for about *one third* of culls in breeding pigs. Apart from the conditions discussed in this section, there are other reasons for lameness, such as general infections like swine erysipelas (see earlier in this chapter) and the inherited susceptibility of certain strains. It has long been apparent that too much emphasis in genetic selection on the growth and carcass quality of the pig can jeopardise the health and vigour of pigs, the strength of the feet and legs being a critical part of this.

Pigs kept outdoors

There has been a significant movement towards keeping adult pigs and breeders outdoors, both as an aid to better health and because of much cheaper capital costs. Housing can be simple and space allowances generous but all outdoor systems require dedicated management and frequent transfer of the pigs on to 'clean' land to prevent disease (Figs 6.4–6.6).

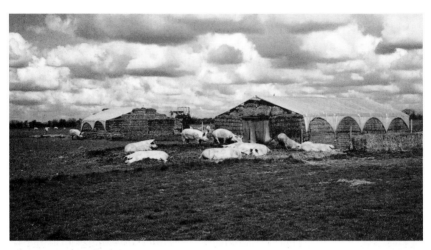

Fig. 6.4   Pigs on free range combined with straw yard accommodation. Such a system is economical in capital cost, healthy, allows generous space allowance and good animal welfare conditions. It does demand copious quantities of good quality straw and dedicated management.

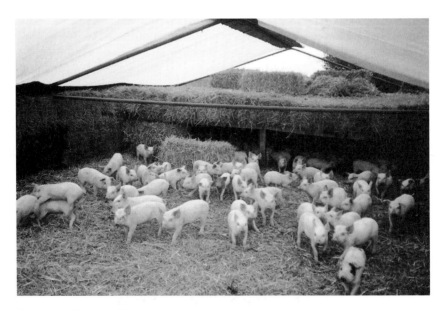

Fig. 6.5   Cheap and healthy pig housing. A group of weaner pigs, about 6 weeks of age, in a strawed yard. The covered area at the rear gives plenty of natural warmth when required and the whole yard is covered with a simple plastic roof.

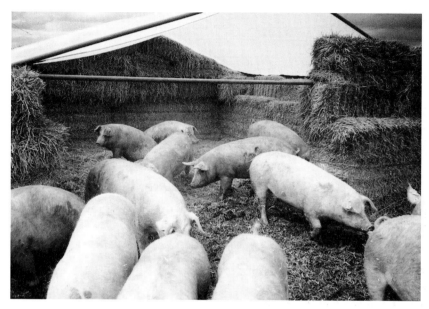

Fig. 6.6 Finishing pigs in healthy, housed accommodation which is deeply strawed, warm and comfortable with a generous space allowance.

Table 6.1 The health of pigs: a summary of diseases, prevention and treatment.

Disease	Prevention	Treatment
Anthrax	(Notifiable in UK) Vaccine. Antiserum	Antiserum. Penicillin
Atrophic rhinitis	Vaccine. Improve environment, especially ventilation. Tylosin. Sulpha drugs	Tylosin. Sulpha drugs
Aujeszky's disease	(Notifiable in UK) Vaccines	None
Bowel oedema	Avoid overfeeding after weaning. Ensure ready access to drinking water or wet feed	Antihistamines. *E. coli* antiserum. Broad-spectrum antibiotics
Clostridial infections	Vaccine. Antiserum	Antiserum. Penicillin. Amoxycillin. Broad-spectrum antibiotics

Table 6.1   Continued

Disease	Prevention	Treatment
E. coli infections	Serum. Vaccines (e.g. Intagen). Appropriate antibiotics	A wide range of antibiotics by injection and oral route, such as amoxicillin, Lincospectin, trimethoprim. Sulphonamides. Framomycin. Neomycin and supportive therapy using minerals, electrolytes and vitamins
Enzootic pneumonia	Consider improving ventilation and reducing numbers of pigs and their stocking density	Broad-spectrum antibiotics in general according to sensitivity test. Prevention by Suvaxyn vaccine
Farrowing fever (metritis, mastitis, agalactia syndrome (MMA))	Improve hygiene of sow and her quarters before and during farrowing	Oxytocin. Oxytetracycline. Chlortetracycline. Amoxycillin.
Greasy pig disease	Ensure soft bedding or good flooring is provided. Fortify vitamin content of rations	Broad-spectrum antibiotics, e.g. Lincospectin, amoxycillin
Leptospirosis	Antiserum. Vaccines. Attend to hygiene and destroy any rodents	Antiserum. Tetracyclines. Streptomycin and broad-spectrum antibiotics
Lice	Clean pens and equipment using disinfectant with insecticides	Deltamethrin
Mange	Clean accommodation and remove badly infected pigs	Phosmet. Diazinon. Bromocyclen and sulphur. Amitraz
Mulberry heart disease	Increase selenium and vitamin content of ration, especially Vitamin E and fat-soluble vitamins	None
Mycotoxicosis	Avoid feed or litter that may contain moulds. Check any doubtful samples	Supportive therapy of vitamins, minerals and electrolytes and antibiotics to prevent secondary infections
Parakeratosis	Zinc must be in the ration at least to a level of 100 ppm	Add zinc sulphate as in Prevention
Piglet anaemia	Iron dextran injections or iron by oral route using pastes, solution or tablets, or by natural access to pasture	Injection of iron dextran solutions and Vitamin B_{12}

Table 6.1   Continued

Disease	Prevention	Treatment
Porcine reproductive and respiratory syndrome (PRRS or 'blue ear' disease)	Isolation of herd as far as possible from all other pigs	Electrolytes. Treat for secondaries with antibiotics and improve nutrition
Roundworm infestation	Enable pigs to be reared without close contact with their dung	Fenbendazole. Tetramisole. Thiabendazole. Piperazine. Dichlorvos
Salmonellosis	(Notifiable in UK) Improve system of management and possibly use vaccines and drugs similar to those given under Treatment	Sulphonamides. Tetracyclines. Lincospectin. Streptomycin. Amoxycillin. Enrofloxacin
'SMEDI' and related virus infections	Often prevented by deliberate early exposure of breeders to infection in a controlled way	Supportive therapy including injection of vitamins, liquids by mouth with electrolytes and broad-spectrum antibiotics to reduce secondary infections
Streptococcal infections	In-feed medication with penicillin	Penicillin. Trimethoprim. Broad-spectrum antibiotics
Swine dysentery	Improve husbandry and management to separate pigs from contact with infected dung. Drugs listed under Treatment may also be used for prevention	Tylosin. Erythromycin. Spiramycin. Tylosin + sulpha drugs. Lincomycin. Lincospectin. Tiamulin
Swine erysipelas	Vaccine. Antiserum	Antiserum. Penicillin or broad-spectrum antibiotics
Swine influenza	Isolation. Low stocking density	Treat for secondaries. Revert to extensive systems
Transmissible gastroenteritis (TGE)	Vaccines available in certain countries	Non-specific supportive therapy and broad-spectrum antibiotics

Chapter 7

The Health of Sheep

Health problems at or near lambing

The health of sheep is dealt with here in the same way as has been done with cattle and pigs, that is on a life-cycle basis and commencing with disease conditions and the maintenance of health at the time of lambing. The first point to stress is the essential need for the highest standard of hygiene at all times. In the life of sheep, lambing is the period of greatest risk from infection; there is almost equal danger to the ewes and their lambs.

Ewes must be carefully observed during lambing to reduce losses due to difficulties in the birth of the lamb (dystocia). Up to 4% of ewes may experience difficulties and if assistance is given the loss can be reduced to about 1%.

It is always difficult to decide when assistance should be given but the general advice is that if no progress is made within 3 hours of the start of lambing the competent shepherd should carry out an examination. He may then find he can readily correct any malpresentation or may decide to call in a veterinary surgeon according to his assessment of the position.

E. coli infection (colibacillosis)

This is perhaps the most serious disease. There are essentially two different types: the enteric and septicaemic forms. Symptoms in the enteric form usually manifest themselves between 1 and 4 days of age and the lamb becomes depressed, shows profuse diarrhoea or dysentery and dies, usually within 24–36 hours of the onset of symptoms. Those affected with the septicaemic form are usually 2–6 weeks old. Affected lambs have a fever and become stiff and uncoordinated in their movements; later they lie down, paddle their legs and become comatose.

The disease usually occurs after a period of lambing due to the 'build-up' of infection that tends to occur during the intensive use of an area. Lambing quarters should not be overused; this can lead to all manner of problems. Nevertheless, it may be possible to prevent the trouble from occurring by injecting a vaccine into the ewes during pregnancy so that the lambs acquire some passive immunity to protect them from the disease during the earlier days of their life. When an outbreak of E. *coli* occurs then a number of treatments can be considered. It is possible to give an antiserum if desired but it is more usual to inject broad-spectrum antibiotics to treat lambs with this worrying condition. If there is evidence of intestinal infection it is also advisable to treat the lambs with an oral dose of antibiotics. Another but quite distinct condition caused by E. *coli* of certain strains is 'watery mouth'. In this disease affected lambs show symptoms very early in life, stop suckling, show marked depression and drool saliva from the mouth in lengthy strings – hence the name of the condition. Such lambs almost invariably die unless they are immediately given supportive fluids, such as electrolyte solutions with the addition of antibiotics and glucose. The most important pre-vantative is to ensure every lamb has its share of colostrum but some E. *coli* vaccines may be helpful.

Navel-ill

This is virtually the same in sheep as in other species. Dirty environmental conditions impede healing of the navel and the infection that may penetrate this point – bacterial in nature – can kill the lamb either in a septicaemic acute way, or more often by leading to general infection of the organs and certain parts of the body, especially the joints. There is only one answer: cleanse the quarters, clean the navel with antiseptic and a dusting of anti-biotic and the troubles should be over. Affected lambs may respond to antibiotic injections if they are administered very quickly after the symptoms are observed.

Mastitis

It is usual for a number of ewes to develop an infection of one or other of the halves of the udder. This is a very damaging disease in ewes which often leads to the complete destruction of the parts affected. It is difficult to know why this condition occurs, although bad hygiene apparently plays its part, but quick treatment with a broad-spectrum antibiotic, given both locally into the teat and by injection, may save the udder and the ewe. Staphylo-coccal, pasturella and clostridial organisms are frequently involved so that gangrene and general tissue destruction can be severe if the disease goes unchecked.

From young lambs to mature sheep

The clostridial diseases

The group of bacteria known as clostridia are spore-forming organisms found almost universally wherever sheep are kept. As soon as the bacteria pass out of the animal's body they form tough spores (or capsules) which make them extremely resistant to destruction. Normally, they may live in the soil for many years. Although we associate the main diseases they cause with sheep, where they tend to transcend all others in importance, they can affect most other livestock and in some cases, man. Their mode of action is to manufacture toxins which make the animal ill or kill it. Under certain circumstances favourable to the bacteria they can and do multiply in large numbers; otherwise the organisms may be present in small numbers and cause no trouble. Clostridia will multiply only in areas where there is no oxygen and they do this in wounds, especially deep ones, in the intestines of animals, or in organs within the body such as the liver. Rather strangely, clostridial diseases tend to most seriously affect animals in very good, thriving condition.

Lamb dysentery

This is caused by a form of clostridium known as *Clostridium perfringens*, Type B. This organism is widespread, like most clostridia, but still tends to be localised in certain areas. The disease occurs in lambs in the first few weeks of life but displays itself in a number of different ways: acute, sub-acute, and chronic forms are described. Whilst the principal symptoms are of bloody diarrhoea (dysentery), the disease may start in a fairly mild way in a flock in the lambing season but gradually increases in severity and intensity as the season continues and will quickly cause many deaths: up to 30% of the flock if it is unchecked.

The first lambs affected may be several weeks old but as the season advances the lambs are affected earlier and eventually as soon as they are born. In many cases no symptoms are seen, the lamb or lambs being found dead, usually overnight. Post-mortem examination shows a very dehydrated carcass and an inflamed and ulcerated small intestine.

Control
As soon as an outbreak occurs, treatment and prevention are achieved successfully by the immediate application of the hyperimmune antiserum. However, to prevent attacks in the future it is much better to vaccinate the ewes. If they are given two vaccinations, the last one being about 1 month

before lambing, they will transfer a strong immunity to the lambs, which will then be safely protected. In succeeding years ewes will need only one additional 'booster' injection.

Pulpy kidney disease

The second of the clostridial diseases that is common in sheep is caused by *Clostridium perfringens* Type D. Symptoms may not be seen, the first sign often being the sudden occurrence of a number of deaths in really good lambs at 2–3 months of age. However, the disease does not only occur at that age, it may occur when store lambs and ewes are put on good pasture in the autumn. It will tend to affect only the best lambs and will also be more likely when animals go on to a better plane of nutrition. The name 'pulpy kidney' is given because on post mortem the kidneys show a high degree of destruction.

Control

As with lamb dysentery the disease can be treated or instant protection is achieved with the antiserum, whilst vaccination of the ewe during pregnancy will give the necessary protection to the lambs for the first weeks of life. However, because a major predisposing cause is the provision of too lush and nutritious a pasture, much can be done to prevent trouble by watching the animals' condition and regulating their nutrition.

Struck

This quite rare condition is caused by a third type of *Clostridium perfringens* Type C and affects lambs over 2 weeks of age but chiefly 1–2 years old. The disease tends to happen after the sheep have been put on improved grazing in winter and spring. It occurs in the UK in Romney Marsh and limited western and northern areas. It can be controlled in the usual way for clostridial disease – that is, remove the cause and treat with antibiotics or antisera.

Blackleg

In this case the clostridia (*Clostridium chauvoei*) do not infect the intestine but the muscles, usually those of the limbs. It appears that after some injury to the body the organisms gain entry and then multiply. The symptoms are caused by toxins destroying muscles and generating gas which causes swelling of the area and a general discoloration and darkening of the skin. It is, in effect, the condition known as *gas gangrene*. It also tends to affect the best sheep and it is the younger ones that are at risk as they have little natural immunity. The disease is similar in nature to blackquarter in cattle (see Chapter 5).

Control
As with other clostridial diseases, vaccines can be given to prevent it. Treatment of affected animals or immediate protection is effective using penicillin injections and/or the specific antiserum.

Braxy

Braxy is caused by *Clostridium septicum*. Usually the first sign is the sudden death of some young sheep in good condition on frosty autumn mornings. The predisposing cause is the eating of frosty food which damages the wall of the abomasum and allows the invasion of the clostridial organisms. Post-mortem signs are of a very inflamed and degenerate abomasal wall. Sometimes some symptoms are seen before death but these are not diagnostic, being those of dullness, inappetence, diarrhoea and incoordination. The most likely age incidence is from 6 to 16 months. The disease tends to be confined to certain areas, especially northern hilly regions. Vaccination is totally effective as a preventive.

Black disease

The symptoms again are sudden death, usually in adult sheep. The organism *Clostridium oedematiens* Type B invades the liver after damage by the liver fluke. It usually occurs in the autumn and early winter when flukes migrate in their largest numbers from the intestine to the liver.

Post-mortem signs are of general degeneration of the body's organs but in particular of the liver, which shows characteristic foci of necrosis.

Control
The same measures are used as in other clostridial diseases. It will also help to prevent black disease if the fluke infestation is controlled.

Tetanus

Tetanus or lockjaw, caused by *Clostridium tetani*, is not the same as other diseases since it does not cause sudden death. In this case the organism finds entry through a wound, which may be an accidental wound or a deliberate one such as castration. The wound heals over and the organism multiplies within this anaerobic atmosphere, producing the toxin which causes nervous symptoms – spasms of muscular contraction, stiffening of the limbs and eventually death.

Control
Control and prevention is along the same lines as for other clostridial diseases. It may also be pointed out that proper attention to injuries with cleansing and treatment will greatly reduce the likelihood of tetanus infection in sheep. As with other of the clostridial diseases, it is beneficial if the sheep are not kept on the same land for too long. Whilst it is true that the sporulating bacteria can exist for a very long time in the soil, resting and cultivation will reduce the numbers and also the risk.

The use of vaccines and sera with clostridial infections

All the clostridial diseases can be countered by the use of sera and vaccines – sera for immediate prevention or treatment, or vaccines to build up an immunity over a period of weeks (see Fig. 7.1). In order to assist the use of the vaccines the pharmaceutical companies have prepared preparations that combine several vaccines together – up to at least eight, covering all the common sheep diseases, are now available. However, it is best not to use these all regardless of need but to choose only those that are entirely necessary. As examples Mallinkrodt manufacture a vaccine, 'Covexin 8', which gives protection against eight clostridial species and Hoechst have a vaccine against seven species of clostridia or a further vaccine which has in addition protection against pasteurella. Initial programmes of vaccination usually require two injections and thereafter booster doses at 6 month or yearly periods.

Respiratory conditions

Pneumonia

Many losses occur from acute pneumonia in sheep and these have undoubtedly been more frequent and more serious in their incidence with the advent of more intensive methods. However, in recent years it is significant that it is *both the acute and chronic* forms which have been increasing.

Acute pneumonia infections, which are especially serious in winter and autumn, are caused by infection with pasteurella bacteria. These organisms are common and normal inhabitants of the respiratory system but manage to generate disease under certain stressful conditions. Such 'triggers' to acute pasteurella infection can be intensification, harmful weather conditions,

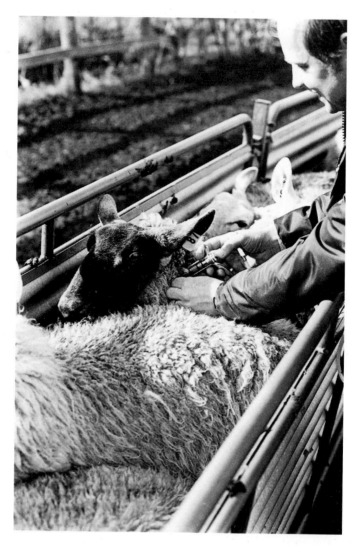

Fig. 7.1   A ewe being vaccinated with a multivalent clostridial infection. Note the way in which the ewes are well controlled in the crush so that the operator carries out the injection easily and without risk of injury to the animals.

transportation under less than ideal conditions, and infestation of the lungs with parasites.

Treatment of pneumonia is best undertaken by the use of antibiotics such as amoxycillin, which have a good activity against pasteurella. Sulphonamide administration is also satisfactory. If problems are anticipated pasteurella vaccine may be administered and this is a wise precaution, particularly in housed sheep where the risk is really very great. It may be emphasised that the environment in housed sheep is nearly always wrong because it is underventilated. I have never seen a sheep house with too much air! The reader is referred to the section on pneumonia in Chapter 5 and in particular the details given of good ventilating practice.

Pulmonary adenomatosis (jaagsiekte)

This is a contagious neoplastic (tumour-forming) disease of the lungs of adult sheep of insidious but continuous development, accompanied by weakness, nasal discharge, laboured breathing and invariably death. It is caused by a slow-acting herpes virus. The only control is by slaughtering infected animals. It does not occur frequently in the UK but is quite common worldwide.

Orf (contagious pustular dermatitis)

Orf, or contagious pustular dermatitis, is a virus infection of sheep which affects the skin, causing vesicles and scabs, especially on the mouth and legs. It may even spread to the inside of the mouth and the genital organs. It can also cause an unpleasant disease in those handling sheep.

Orf is caused by a virus and older animals develop an immunity after infection. Thus the infection is found mostly in young stock. It can have only a mild effect in the older lamb but is extremely serious in the younger animal and can even cause death. A good live virus vaccine is available and, if orf is a common and serious problem in a stock, is best used in an attempt not only to control but eventually to eliminate the trouble altogether.

Deficiency conditions

Swayback (enzootic ataxia)

Swayback is one of the best known mineral deficiency diseases. It affects the nervous system of young lambs either at birth or a week or two thereafter. The symptoms are of incoordination and paralysis of the limbs of the body due to degeneration of the nerve cells in the brain and spinal column; it is associated with a low level of copper in the blood and tissues of the lambs and ewes. The basic cause of the disease is a deficiency of copper, this element being essential for the formation of enzymes for the construction of nervous tissue. The critical level of copper necessary for the proper development of nervous tissue is 5 ppm. In swayback areas levels of copper are generally well below this. The disease also tends to occur at its worst when the pasture is very lush and weather conditions have been particularly favourable to good growth.

Blood copper levels in swayback-affected lambs are very low, as indeed they are in the ewes, but the strange fact is that only a proportion of lambs born to ewes with low levels of copper actually have swayback. Thus the whole reason for this disease is not fully understood. However, in order to prevent the disease, it is necessary to supplement the copper intake of the pregnant ewe. Mineral mixtures need to be given by some means or another. Individual dosing or the use of long-acting injectables are further ways of providing the copper and have the merit that they do provide a known dose to every ewe. Adult ewes require an average daily intake of 5–10 mg of copper as an adequate allowance. Mineral block mixtures containing 0.5% copper sulphate are satisfactory. Alternatively diet supplementation with 0.2 g of copper sulphate fed weekly to each sheep would be adequate.

Top dressing of the pasture is not advised as it is wasteful, inexact and may give rise to toxicity. Copper toxicity is a very serious condition and sheep are the most susceptible of farm animals to this condition; they accumulate copper quite slowly before symptoms appear. Cases have always tended to occur in housed sheep fed diets that are too rich in copper.

Pine (pining)

Pine is a disease of sheep which leads to wasting and is caused by a deficiency of cobalmin, alternatively known as Vitamin B_{12}. However, the deficiency is not a straightforward deficiency. Cobalmin is an essential vitamin which is synthesised by the bacteria which are present in the sheep's stomach, but in order that this can take place there must be sufficient cobalt in the diet as cobalt is an essential constituent of this vitamin.

Lack of cobalt may be a simple deficiency of the element or there may be such a preponderance of calcium that the cobalt is chemically tied to this and is not available in sufficient amounts for absorption. In either case it is a disease of great economic importance. A simple way of preventing pining is to add a supplement which has been enriched with cobalt to the normal concentrate feed. Animals may also be dosed individually but this is rather tiresome because it must be done on several occasions, indeed once weekly if necessary. The cobalt 'bullet' is thus the best treatment since it is released gradually over a long period (see also Chapter 5). One 'bullet' is usually sufficient for 12 months and each 5 g 'bullet' contains 90% cobalt oxide. Some 'bullets' are eliminated by the sheep so it is still necessary to watch their condition closely and re-dose as soon as this is apparent. The pasture may also be treated and this is done quite easily by spreading about 2 kg of cobalt sulphate per acre about every 5 years.

Rickets

Rickets – a condition of poor bone construction when the calcification fails to take place efficiently – is sometimes seen in lambs. Proper formation of bones takes place when there is a sufficient quantity and balance of the minerals calcium and phosphorus, together with Vitamin D. Unless all these minerals are adequately provided, rickets occurs. It is not easy to explain how lambs can suffer from serious deficiencies under normal husbandry conditions but injections of Vitamin D are usually successful in arresting the problem.

Internal parasites of sheep

The three main types of internal parasites that infest sheep are tapeworms, flatworms (represented by the liver fluke), and roundworms (which infest both the intestines and the lungs).

Tapeworms

Tapeworms require an intermediate host, as well as sheep, for their existence. The adult tapeworm lives in the sheep's intestines where it lays eggs which pass out in the dung on to the pasture and further development can occur only if it is picked up by the intermediate host. The sheep is host to only one adult tapeworm, the 'milkworm' which infests mainly suckling lambs. The secondary host is a small pasture mite; lambs become infested when they consume the mites accidentally when grazing.

It is thought improbable that these tapeworms do very much harm unless the infestation is a very heavy one, in which case it is necessary to treat the lambs. There is no way of effectively getting rid of the secondary host.

Sheep may also be infested with a number of bladder worms, infestation being picked up on grazing contaminated with the droppings of dogs and foxes which carry the adult tapeworms in their intestines. These bladder worms occur as thin-walled, fluid-filled bladders, usually up to 50 mm in diameter and which are found among the intestines, in the lung and liver and in the nervous system. Although of little harm to sheep, two are also found in man and are a public health concern. Whilst they are relatively uncommon, all raw sheep offal and carcasses should be carefully disposed of to prevent infestation of dogs and foxes.

Liver fluke

Liver fluke is a serious problem in many parts of the world in wet years and infestations in Great Britain are most serious in the wetter parts of the country. It has a two-host life-cycle, the adults living in the bile ducts of the liver in sheep, cattle and other animals and the intermediate younger stages in a snail. The snail can exist only in areas where the soil is saturated with moisture for considerable periods, although it is not found naturally in running water or ponds. In dry periods or in winter it tends to burrow into the mud and can survive in the inactive state for a considerable time.

Hatching and development of fluke eggs is restricted by the climatic temperature and humidity requirements to the period from May to September, coinciding with the season of activity of the snail. When hatched the larvae must find and penetrate a snail within about 24 hours. Within the snail a number of developmental stages occur, the final form leaving the snail and attaching to vegetation and forming a protective capsule. This stage is infective to sheep and attacks the liver, where it wanders in the tissue for 2–3 months and then settles into the bile ducts. Acute fluke disease occurs during the migration of the larvae in the liver in heavy infestation and the chronic disease occurs some months later as the adult flukes cause thickening of the bile ducts and they also interfere with normal liver function. The total period from egg to adult is 5–6 months, producing one generation of flukes each year, thus explaining the incidence of the acute disease in the spring and chronic disease in the autumn. The economic importance of fluke losses varies considerably from year to year but it is important to institute some control measures in areas where the disease is common. The first thing to do is to treat the sheep with appropriate medicines, such as diamphenethide; secondly measures should be taken to prevent the sheep becoming infected by either isolating them from the area of the snails or by destroying the snails. If the area can be drained more efficiently, that will also serve a very useful purpose. Treatment of land to rid it of snails includes the use of copper sulphate solution and sodium pentachlorophenate.

One of the difficulties with fluke control has been that it is difficult to justify taking expensive control measures when the likelihood of infection only occurs every few years. However, it is now known that an infection can be predicted, depending on the rainfall that occurred in late winter and spring; thus control can be put in operation just at the time it is appropriate.

Roundworms of sheep

At least ten species of roundworms (nematodes) cause parasitic gastroenteritis (or nematode gastroenteritis), which is considered the most economically serious cause of loss in sheep. Heavy infestations are disastrous but even light ones can cause a great loss of productivity. Principal worms are *Haemonchus contortus, Ostertagia circumcincta, Trichostrongylus axei, Nematodirus spathiger, Trichuris ovis* and *Oesophagostomum columbianum.*

In the control measures, attention is directed principally to animals in the first year of life as this is the time when they are severely affected. The older sheep usually develop a degree of resistance to infection.

The parasitic roundworms do not multiply in the sheep, and their numbers are increased only by the intake of fresh infection. The degree of infection therefore depends on the build-up of the worm burden in the pasture with the eggs of the worms and the frequency of the contact between the grazing animal and this contaminated pasture. Control is tackled in two ways: firstly by treatment of the animal to eliminate the worm burden, and secondly by pasture and flock management to minimise infection.

Medicines that are used to control the infections must have a wide spectrum of safety and yet be highly effective. Recently some very good products have emerged, the benzimiadoles, the imidazothiazoles, the tetrahydropyrimidines and organophosphorus preparations, which are effective against all intestinal stages of the worm. They clear out the worms effectively but of course do not prevent reinfestation. This is achieved by suitable pasture management which is based on rotational grazing, allowing up to a week on pasture then closing it for 3 weeks. This is because eggs take about a week to become effective, and if they do not find a host most perish within 4 weeks.

Sheep may also be affected by lungworms and the reader is referred to Chapter 5 for a description of the similar condition in cattle.

External parasites

It is difficult to exaggerate the danger to sheep of the various species of external parasites; these include insects, mites and ticks which show con- siderable similarities in their physiology and susceptibility to chemicals and can really be treated as a group. These parasites can only be effectively dealt with when they are actually on the animal. The easiest to kill are those which spend their whole time on the sheep – the mites, lice and keds – and which cannot survive off the host for more than a couple of weeks. This group is effectively controlled by a single whole-body treatment with a preparation which is lethal to adults and young stages and persistent enough to kill the larvae as they hatch from resistant eggs, or by repeated use of a material which kills the adult only. This was the basis for the traditional double-dipping and single-dipping regulations which controlled sheep scab, which is caused by the psoroptic mange parasite (Fig. 7.2).

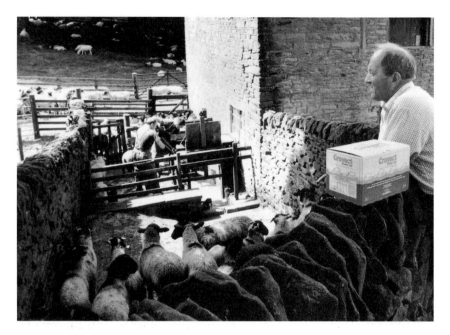

Fig. 7.2   Sheep dipping in progress on a farm in the Lake District. Although of a simple, traditional design the arrangement ensures that the sheep can be handled easily and the slope of the ground assists in achieving good drainage.

The compulsory treatment of all suspected cases led at one time to the eradication of sheep scab in the British Isles once the highly effective DDT and BHC preparations (now superseded) became available.

The sheep scab treatment also effectively controlled lice and keds, but now lice are frequently resistant to the common insectides. The *blowfly*, in comparison with the other external parasites, completes only one fairly short stage of its development on the sheep and is thus open to attack by an insecticide for only a short time. Larvae hatch rapidly and feed on the skin and tissues for several days, then they fall on to the herbage and form the resting stage, known as the pupa, from which the adult fly emerges several weeks later. The flies' breeding activity extends from about May to September and several generations will emerge during that time.

Thus the problems of blowfly control are the limited period in which it is possible to attack the parasite on the animal, the repeated infestation and the very severe damage done by the larvae. However, modern organophosphorus compounds and carbamate mixtures are quite effective if properly applied. Whole body dipping is really the most satisfactory method; it is better than spraying, which is not thorough in its penetration.

The problem of fly-strike requires additional measures to be effective. All cases of scour should be treated and wounds should be dressed immediately.

Any weakness of an area attracts the flies and can be a contributing cause of the breakdown of a control programme.

In the north of England and in Scotland a very nasty problem, the *headfly*, has recently emerged. This fly, which is very similar to the housefly, feeds on the fluid from the eyes, nose and mouth of sheep. As a result of the irritation the sheep rub their heads against fences and walls causing wounds which make them even more attractive to the unwelcome attention of the headfly. The result of this disturbance is a very restless animal and considerable economic loss.

The *sheep tick* spends even less of its life actually on the animal. It attaches itself only for a relatively few days during its 3 year cycle of development, the rest of the time being spent on the pasture where it requires a high moisture level for prolonged survival and so infestation is common in rough pasture, particularly woodland. The principal active time is in the spring and early summer, with another period of activity in the moist time of autumn. Most ticks, therefore, are only able to be destroyed over these two relatively short periods, each of about 3 weeks' duration. The preparation that is used must therefore be highly active against all the developmental ages and should protect the sheep over a period of about 2 months. Some note should be given to the other methods of control involving the improvement of pasture so that it is less attractive to the tick.

Sheep scab, the commonly used name for a mange in sheep is caused by the psoroptic mange parasite. This mange parasite can invade all parts of the body that are covered with wool, as well as the ears. The total effect is extremely damaging, which is the reason for the disease being notifiable. Although at one time it was eliminated from sheep in the UK it has now returned. The mite in its progress in the skin causes injuries and serum oozes out on which it feeds; the wounds develop scabs after a time, hence the name 'sheep scab'. The poison produced by the mite causes intense irritation so the sheep rubs and scratches itself endlessly, the skin becomes thickened and ulcerated and the wool is detached and the sheep looks increasingly ill.

Treatment is instituted by a dipping of the sheep with approved materials. Prevention is also achieved by a regular dipping procedure. Excellent dips are produced which in one treatment give a long-term, persistent (residual) effect. Only approved dips should be used, such as those based on flumethrin, diazinon, cypermethrin and amitraz.

Great care is required in the actual procedure of dipping sheep. The following precautions are essential. Sheep should not be dipped for 1 month after service and great care should be taken with pregnant ewes at other times. Sheep should be offered water to drink before they are dipped to help prevent them drinking the dip, and the dip should be chosen to prevent any damage to the wool. The sheep should be rested before dipping and must be drained of dip before being turned out to pasture again. The dip itself must be disposed of safely after use to prevent any contamination of water courses. Above all, those carrying out the dipping should be trained and should wear protective clothing and all those measures advised officially and on the literature accompanying the dip must be taken. Organophosporus compounds which are so successful as dips may be a health risk to those doing the dipping unless these precautions are heeded.

Other forms of mange do occur in sheep, for example, sarcoptic mange, but this is usually only on the head, and chorioptic mange, which is in the pastern and interdigital space of the feet. None of these forms are as bad as the psoroptic mange mite.

Infections of mature sheep

Scrapie

Scrapie is caused by an organism known as a prion and details of the condition and its close affinity to BSE can be found in Chapter 4. The disease has an immensely protracted incubation period and even after the symptoms develop it may take as much as 6 months for death – which is inevitable – to take place.

The organism affects the nervous system, causing alternating periods of lethargy and excitability. As the disease progresses the sheep become unable to control their hindquarters and then develop a severe itchiness which makes the sheep bite frantically at the area of irritation, or rub furiously against posts or other protuberances, which can then result in a very bedraggled fleece and sore, raw places. The disease affects some breeds more than others; indeed some strains seem to be completely resistant to the disease so that breeding from resistant strains offers a method of eliminating the infection.

The long incubation period of up to 3 years has made research a problem but generally the condition occurs sporadically with just a limited proportion of sheep being affected. Control is also difficult, no treatment is of any use and all sheep that are infected will die.

All infected sheep should be slaughtered; in fact, to deal with the disease correctly the ancestors and progeny should be slaughtered as well. A technique that has been used successfully to eliminate scrapie from a flock is to slaughter all the infected animals and then to take replacement ewe lambs only from mature mothers at their third or later lambings. Scrapie is rarely seen in sheep over 5 years of age. Unfortunately, because of the long incubation period it is very difficult ever to know when or if a flock is free of the disease; this makes it difficult to see how the disease can ever be completely eradicated.

Johne's disease

This condition in sheep is similar to that in cattle (see Chapter 5). The disease organism, *Mycobacterium johnei*, causes a chronic wasting condition of older sheep accompanied by a characteristically foetid form of scour. Lambs pick up the infection when they are very young from infected pasture, although no symptoms are seen at this time. It is later in life, perhaps as long as 3 years, and – under the stress of poor management, nutrition or housing that the condition becomes apparent. There is no cure and affected sheep must be culled. It is possible to protect sheep with a vaccine but it is more important to try to remove the opportunities for infection of the young lambs.

Foot rot

This remains one of the biggest causes of serious economic loss in sheep everywhere. It is primarily caused by the bacterium *Fusiformis nodosus* and occurs widely if not properly controlled. It spreads from sheep to sheep via infected soil, but the bacteria do not live many days in the soil. The harbourers of infection are, in fact, the sheep with bad feet in which the organism can survive indefinitely. The conditions that favour the spread of infection are wet weather and soil when the feet are softened and the organisms released to invade other feet through any injured part.

Control of foot rot

Control programmes must be instituted because it has been well established that infection has a profound effect on profitability. A suitable programme will make use of the following facts:

- ❏ The organism only infects sheep
- ❏ It can only survive outside the sheep for about 2 weeks
- ❏ Treatment can be very effective provided the areas of the feet which harbour infection are exposed

Firstly, all feet must be inspected and trimmed and all bad cases showing inflamed areas should be separated. Those with very badly shaped feet may be symptomless carriers and should also be separated. All healthy sheep are then walked through a foot bath which contains a 5–10% solution of formalin. Contact with the formalin should last at least 1 minute. After this the sheep are put on to clean concrete for an hour or so then on to pasture which has had no sheep on it for some weeks.

Secondly, those with affected feet must be handled individually. All the damaged, separated horn should be carefully pared away so that the inflamed and infected tissue is exposed to the air and to treatment. During paring great care must be taken not to damage the feet by cutting the living tissue.

The foot, having been prepared in this way, is then treated with a suitable preparation. This may be 10% formalin, but suitable antibiotic preparations are to be preferred as they have a gentle, more specific action. Then, the treated group should be kept entirely separate from the healthy animals so that the former can be handled and retreated at something like weekly intervals. After this period the sheep can then rejoin the main flock, but any that seem incurable are best culled as they may be a constant source of reinfection and very costly to maintain. It is as well to try and choose a suitable period to carry out this eradication programme and the driest summer weather is best.

The metabolic diseases of sheep

There are three important metabolic diseases of sheep: pregnancy toxaemia (or twin lamb disease), milk fever (lambing sickness) and hypomagnesaemia (grass staggers).

Pregnancy toxaemia (twin lamb disease)

This is a disease of ewes which affects them in the last few weeks of pregnancy and nearly always in ewes which are carrying more than one lamb. First symptoms are of incoordination but the affected ewes quickly become totally recumbent and comatose and will invariably die unless treated.

The condition to some extent is due to excessive demands being made on the ewes' metabolism when associated with insufficient nutrition. Afflicted ewes may need injections of intravenous glucose solution together with dosing with glycerine and/or glucose solutions. However, most of the effort should go into prevention. The important and indeed essential requirement is that during the last 6 weeks of pregnancy the ewe should be given a diet which is low in fibre, nutritious and easily digested. The nutritional problem is often exacerbated by the bad conditions which may face the ewes in the winter months, diverting the feed being given from building up strength to keeping the ewe alive in the face of the cold. As with most metabolic disorders, the condition is not simply a deficiency and it appears to be especially likely to occur if there is some stress, be it environmental or nutritional, late in pregnancy (see also Chapter 5).

Milk fever (lambing sickness)

This is virtually the same as in the dairy cow with a serious fall of blood calcium occurring soon after lambing and associated with the rapid production of milk by the ewe. The symptoms are depression and coma. Treatment is an immediate injection of calcium borogluconate given either intravenously or subcutaneously.

Hypomagnesaemia (grass staggers)

This is caused by a low level of magnesium in the blood, the effect usually being sudden death without any symptoms. Alternatively, there may be some symptoms of hyperexcitability which eventually lead to coma and death. The problem usually occurs soon after lambing. The highest incidence is in ewes on chalk soil and during cold and wet weather. It is a condition associated with intensive husbandry and with rather excessively lush pasture. The treatment is to administer an injection of a magnesium solution as quickly as possible.

Prevention is not easy. The cause of the problem is, as with cattle, a shortage of magnesium which has to be provided one way or another. Supplementary feeding with a mixture of molasses and magnesium using a special feeder is good, the molasses making an unpalatable magnesium mixture into a palatable one. The best method, however, it to use a magnesium 'bullet'. This consists of a heavy magnesium-rich ball or 'bullet' which is given to the ewe and which lodges in the reticulum. The magnesium is absorbed over a number of weeks and will safely carry the ewe over the danger period.

Diseases causing abortions

There are several diseases – viral, bacterial and parasitic – that lead to abortions and their economic importance can be very great. It should also be noted that in sheep, as in all animals, any disease that has a serious generalised effect during pregnancy can lead to abortion.

Enzootic abortion

This is caused by a chlamydial organism and tends to be common in certain well-defined areas; in the UK it is especially prevalent in north-east England and south-east Scotland. The infection is usually introduced into a flock by a 'carrier' which releases a great amount of infected material when it aborts.

This infects the ewe lambs which will not abort the first season but will abort in the second. After abortion they are then immune but young sheep and bought-in animals will continue to become infected.

There is no specific treatment for infected animals but it is good policy to isolate the ewes which have aborted for the period when they may be discharging infected material. Thereafter a policy of vaccination may need to be instituted. Good vaccines are available and will protect the non-infected animals satisfactorily: one administration being sufficient for life.

Salmonellosis

Salmonellosis abortion is an acute and contagious condition caused by the bacterium *Salmonella abortus ovis*, and which can also be caused by non-specific salmonellae, such as *S. typhimurium* and *S. dublin*. It is a condition that is present in virtually all sheep-rearing countries and tends to cause abortions late in pregnancy. The disease does not give rise to specific symptoms – clinically it can be indistinguishable from other causes of abortion – and it is thus imperative to seek professional advice, including a laboratory examination, to be certain of the agent. Once the cause is known measures of control can be instituted, including antibiotics or chemotherapy, vaccination and hygienic measures.

Vibriosis

Vibriosis abortion, caused by *Vibrio foetus*, is another bacterial cause of abortion which, like salmonella infections, causes late abortions. There is no specific treatment but vaccines are available to control the condition.

Brucella

Brucella species of bacteria can also cause abortion in sheep, the effects being the same as in cattle. *Brucella abortus, Brucella mellitensis* and *Brucella ovis* are all capable of causing the problems. After positive diagnosis, control relies on hygiene and vaccination.

Toxoplasmosis

There is also a parasitic cause of abortion in sheep which is due to a toxoplasma: *Toxoplasma gondii*. With this disease it is suggested the best course in an infected flock is to mix infected ewes with non-pregnant ones to stimulate natural immunity before pregnancy, but this is only a partially satisfactory approach.

The notifiable diseases of anthrax and foot and mouth disease also occur in sheep and the reader is referred to Chapter 5 for a full discussion of these.

Table 7.1 The health of sheep: a summary of diseases, prevention and treatment.

Disease	Prevention	Treatment
Black disease	Specific antiserum and vaccine. Avoid fluke-infested pastures	Antibiotics, e.g. amoxycillin and penicillin preparations and wide-spectrum antibiotics generally
Blackleg	Specific antiserum and vaccines	Amoxycillin antiserum, broad-spectrum antibiotics
Braxy	Specific antiserum and vaccines. Frosted food predisposes to infection	Amoxycillin and antiserum or other broad-spectrum antibiotics
Brucellosis	Specific vaccines	Remove all infected animals from the flock
E coli (colibacillosis)	Improved hygiene or new quarters. Antiserum or vaccines	Antiserum. Broad-spectrum antibiotics, e.g. amoxycillin. Supportive fluid therapy
Enzootic abortion	Vaccination	Broad-spectrum antibiotics will limit secondary infection if necessary
Foot rot	Vaccination and careful attention to feet by trimming, and foot baths of zinc sulphate or formalin	As prevention, together with local antibiotic preparations, such as oxytetracycline
Hypomagnesaemia	Magnesium preparations in food or 'licks'. Magnesium 'bullets'	Intravenous magnesium solution
Lamb dysentery	Specific antisera and vaccines	Antiserum, supportive fluid therapy and antibiotics, such as amoxycillin
Liver fluke	Attention to land drainage; destroy snails, the secondary hosts	Diamphenethide, closantel, triclabendazole and other anthelmintics
Mastitis	Improve hygiene	Inject antibiotic appropriate to infection and also administer via teat
Milk fever	Administration of minerals including calcium by oral route or Vitamin D by injection	Calcium borogluconate injections

Table 7.1   Continued

Disease	Prevention	Treatment
Navel-ill	Improve hygiene of lambing quarters. Dress navel with antiseptic at birth	Inject antibiotics with a broad-spectrum of activity
Orf	Specific vaccine	Isolate and treat affected areas with antiseptics and antibiotics
Pining	Dressing pasture with cobalt salt	Dosing with cobalt chloride or administration of cobalt 'bullet'
Pneumonia	Improve environment in housed sheep. Improve nutrition in all cases	Antisera. Vaccines. Sulpha drugs. Antibiotics, e.g. amoxycillin
Pregnancy toxaemia	Improved nutrition in pregnancy	Glycerine. Glucose. Molasses
Pulpy kidney disease	Antiserum and vaccines	Antiserum and penicillin or broad-spectrum antibiotics by injection
Rickets	Improved provision of minerals and vitamins	Vitamin D by injection and minerals
Roundworms	Improved pasture management to prevent infection and especially removal of lambs from contact with infected ground	Levamisole. Febantel. Ricobendazole, benzimidazole. Thiothanate
Salmonellosis	Vaccination where appropriate. Rigid hygiene	Antibiotics, e.g. ampicillin
Sheep scab	Rigid dipping of all sheep	Use only approved dip. Dips include flumethrin, diazinon, cypermethrin, amitraz
Swayback	Administrations of copper preparations to ewes in pregnancy	None
Tetanus	Antitoxin. Vaccine	Antiserum. Antitoxin. Hexamine
Vibriosis	Vaccination	Broad-spectrum antibiotics
Watery mouth	Colostrum and *E. coli* vaccine	Electrolyte fluids, glucose and broad-spectrum antibiotics

Chapter 8

The Health of Poultry

The chick

The day-old chick is especially susceptible to every form of stress and the environmental conditions must be accurately maintained to avoid either chilling or overheating. Since most birds are now kept together in substantial numbers, unless sophisticated environmental control systems (Figs. 8.1 and 8.2) are used it is almost impossible to provide an optimal and uniform environment and whilst the conditions required by the chick are well known, the ability of the housing to provide them properly is often lacking. Thus there may be almost immediate losses from chilling in certain areas of a house, but in general the losses in the chicks in the first 4 or 5 days of life are after-effects of the management and health of the breeders or the management and hygiene of the hatchery.

Yolk-sac infection

This is called 'mushy chick' disease, omphalitis or navel infection, and is undoubtedly the commonest of all conditions causing early mortality. The signs soon show themselves – the chicks so affected are usually abnormal when placed in the brooder house but make no progress and most deaths occur about 36–72 hours after placement. Examination of the chick shows a 'blown-up' abdomen, a wet or scabby navel and a very offensive odour which is virtually diagnostic. If the abdomen is opened, it will be seen that the yolk sac is not absorbed but is filled with discoloured fluid, often brown and infection may have spread throughout the abdominal cavity. The infective agents that cause the disease are bacteria and *Escherichia coli* is frequently the main one involved.

The disease may be due to many different reasons, ranging from mismanagement or bad hygiene in the breeder flocks, to poor hatchery standards and inefficiency in the control of the incubator or hatchery.

There is usually a much bigger incidence of the disease in chicks hatched towards the end of winter or in early spring when the health and condition of the breeding flocks are usually at their poorest. No treatment will save

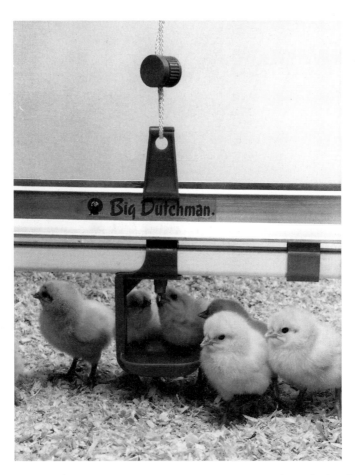

Fig. 8.1 'Nipple drinkers' are widely used for chickens in place of other forms as they are more hygienic and cause less wastage and wetting of litter (courtesy of Big Dutchman).

those chicks affected but it is advisable to treat affected flocks since it may help to limit the spread of infection. The infected birds may release enormous numbers of pathogenic organisms into the environment so the following measures may be logically applied. The warmth of the house should be increased to assist the birds' resistance to infection and help to prevent huddling. Tests should be carried out in the laboratory to establish which organisms are involved and which treatment would be most appropriate. The drinking water should then be medicated with a vitamin and antibiotic mixture. All abnormal chicks should be culled. Careful investigation should be made of the hatchery or breeding organisation as to the likely cause. It is of great importance to do this and trace the source of the disease; if the

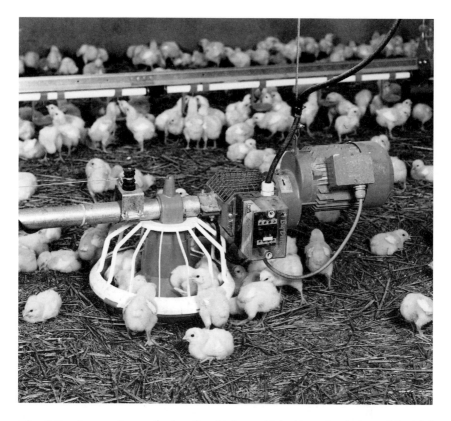

Fig. 8.2   Automatic pan feeders for chicken which allow circulation of the birds around them, favouring good litter conditions (courtesy of Big Dutchman).

breeding management is not informed it may be unaware of the problem and obviously no measures will be taken to stop it. It is quite usual practice in broiler chicks and sometimes in other chicks being reared to include a medicine at a prophylactic level during the first 10 days of life. Examples of the medicines used include potentiated sulphonamides, neomycin, linco-mycin and tetracyclines.

Aspergillosis (or brooder pneumonia)

This is the most important but by no means the only disease of poultry caused by a fungus and leads to early death in chicks. The fungus, usually *Apergillus fumigatus*, is one which occurs widely on farms and in the countryside and can therefore readily contaminate hatching eggs. In its natural environment the fungus needs mouldy, damp conditions in which the moisture content is more than 20% – so it can be common, for example, if breeders are kept on damp litter or there is damp and dirty material in the nests. Hatching eggs can pick up the fungus in the nests or on the litter itself quite readily and the pathogen will then be taken through to the hatchery. If infection enters the hatchery and the fungus is not destroyed by fumigation, an almost explosive incidence can occur in the chicks and mortalities during the first few days of life may vary from a few up to 50% or even more on occasion. Alternatively the chicks themselves can pick up infection from damp and mouldy litter used as their bedding.

The signs of infection are of pneumonia, the chicks gasping and struggling for breath with their mouths open. Post-morten findings are of tiny yellowish-green nodules with a green furry extrusion in the lungs, bronchi, trachea and visceria, whilst the air sacs may be covered with thick yellow exudate. A laboratory will identify the fungus definitely; a sure diagnosis cannot be made by the naked eye or from the symptoms, which may be similar to other diseases.

There is no specific treatment. If outbreaks occur in chicks they provide an important warning that there are serious errors in hygiene and/or management, and it is vital that the areas of infection are located so that remedial steps can be taken. Control measures will include a culling of affected chicks, a more thorough disinfection of housing and equipment, removal of unsuitable litter or nesting material, and better cleaning and fumigation of hatching eggs and equipment and the hatchery. There has been a recent upsurge in aspergillosis due to the more frequent use of chopped straw as the litter in broiler and other poultry houses. The danger is present only if the straw becomes wet, with a more than 20% moisture content.

Salmonellosis

The group of bacteria known as salmonella is world-wide and one of the greatest causes of losses in poultry on a world scale. In many countries, including the UK, prolonged control measures have nowadays led to few losses in poultry due to salmonellosis. It must be stressed that overriding emphasis is now attached to an attempt – which may well be achieved before long – to eradicate salmonella diseases altogether from our birds because certain species of the bacteria are a principal cause of food poisoning in man. It will be appreciated that under intensive conditions there is an extra risk of contagion taking hold of many birds at one time, so it is highly desirable that all possible sources of infection are removed. A few areas of the world – notably Scandinavia – have been able to rid themselves of salmonella infections in animals and man.

Types of salmonella infection

There are two forms of salmonella species which are specific to poultry; these are *Salmonella pullorum* and *Salmonella gallinarum*. The former, perhaps the oldest of all diseases diagnosed in poultry, used to be called bacillary white diarrhoea (BWD), whilst *S. gallinarum* is commonly called fowl typhoid. In addition there are those diseases in poultry caused by other salmonella and coming under the general title of salmonellosis or sometimes termed avian paratyphoid. There are many different forms – at least 200 types of salmonella have been found in poultry – but the most important are *S. enteriditis* and *S. typhimurium* which can be highly pathogenic to poultry and man.

Symptoms

The symptoms of the various forms of salmonella infection vary considerably. Mortalities are extremely variable, ranging from no more than 1 or 2% up to as much as 50% or even more. If chicks, for example, are infected with pullorum disease via the infected hen and thereby spread through the hatchery, signs of illness will occur within a matter of hours of hatching. In cases where the infection is light and the environment and husbandry good, the losses can be modest but early losses from salmonella infection more usually run at between 10 and 20% and may extend over 2 weeks. Early on in life chicks usually die quickly with few symptoms but as the disease proceeds, symptoms progressively appear of huddling, inappetence, constant cheeping, a swollen abdomen and white diarrhoea. There are also chronic cases in which numbers of chicks are stunted, scour, and experience lameness due to swollen joints. These symptoms are much the same for all forms of salmonella infection in chicks and growing birds and it is quite impossible from these symptoms to distinguish either which form of salmonella is present or indeed whether it is a salmonella disease at all.

In the adult, acute salmonella infection is typically that known as *fowl typhoid*, due to *Salmonella gallinarum*. Signs that would lead to suspecting an attack would be when a number of birds scour with greenish-yellow and evil-smelling droppings, have a greatly increased thirst, show very pale (anaemic) head parts and there are also a number of sudden deaths. As mortality may go as high as 75%, with 50% being common, this is a disease which is hardly likely to be missed.

Post-mortem signs in the chick are not diagnostic but are at least strongly suspicious. If the bird dies at the hyper-acute stage the signs are few, apart from congestion of internal organs, especially the liver and lungs. In later cases, where the infection is not acute or sub-acute, the liver and other internal organs show characteristic yellowish nodules and the caecal tubes often contain semi-solid yellow 'casts'. The yolk sac may likewise be filled with a pus-like 'sludge'. In the adult, the post-mortem signs in pullorum or gallinarum infection are similar and especially associated with the ovary in which the ovules are grossly misshapen and the contents are also abnormal. Other internal organs may be infected, including the heart which shows inflammation of the membranes around it (pericarditis). These generally diagnostic symptoms in the adult are only rarely seen with the other forms of salmonella.

The control of salmonella infections

With pullorum and gallinarum infections, simple and rapid on the spot blood tests have been in use for many years and can detect carriers with great accuracy. These tests have been enormously successful since they enable immediate removal of the carrier birds from a flock. Thus the two diseases caused by *Salmonella pullorum* and *S. gallinarum* have been controlled with great success in many countries, including the UK. Under these circumstances only a few isolated cases turn up from time to time detected by the blood tests and regular testing may be necessary only on the foundation breeding stock.

Unfortunately the position with regard to other types of salmonella is entirely different and somewhat confusing. There are some 200 different serotypes that have been isolated from poultry. A few can be quite devastating in their effect, such as *Salmonella typhimurium* and *Salmonella enteriditis*, others are mild or cause no symptoms at all. In every case infection may spread to other livestock or man. It is probable, however, that the main risk is not that the poultry will infect other forms of life, but that other livestock will infect poultry!

In general the symptoms of salmonella infection in chicks are similar to those seen in pullorum disease and indeed it is only possible to distinguish the cause by laboratory examination. Post-mortem lesions do not enable more than suspicions to be raised, although there is always the likely involvement of the liver, which is usually enlarged and congested in salmonella victims.

Because of the great value of attempting to eliminate salmonellosis from poultry, many countries, including the UK, have comprehensive legislation that requires compulsory notification of salmonella infections to the authorities. When flocks are found to be 'positive' to those salmonella serotypes which can have serious human health implications a number of measures can be enforced. Depending on the type of birds involved these, will include procedures ranging from compulsory slaughter of the flock, mandatory administration of approved medicines, and isolation of the premises and supervised and monitored hygienic procedures.

Salmonella eradication is important for several reasons. A number of the salmonellae which infect poultry can be serious causes of food poisoning in man and it is therefore of great public health importance that birds entering the processing plant, in particular, are clear of salmonella either from obvious clinical infections or as symptomless carriers of the disease organisms.

Salmonella in poultry flocks originates from a number of sources. It may come from foodstuffs, especially the animal protein element. In order to control the entry of salmonella infection via foodstuffs it is necessary for all protein foods of animal source, or other feeds that could be contaminated, to be either heat or chemically treated before they are used. There is now a very successful vaccine to prevent *Salmonella enteritidis* and it is anticipated that additional salmonella vaccines will soon be made.

Gumboro disease (infectious bursal disease)

This is an extremely serious virus infection which occurs in most areas of the world. It was first reported in 1962 in the USA and very soon afterwards appeared in the UK and Western Europe. The symptoms of the disease generally first show as an acute infection of sudden onset in young chicks, mostly broilers, then a quick peak of mortality followed by a return to normality which leaves a substantial number of birds stunted in their growth and very unproductive. Affected chicks show anorexia, depression, huddling, ruffled feathers, vent pecking, diarrhoea, trembling and incoordination. The most significant post-morten sign is an extreme inflammation of the bursa of Fabricius (Fig. 8.3) which will be greatly enlarged and oedematous. After the inflammatory period it becomes small and shrivelled.

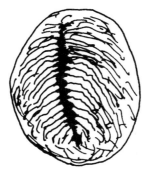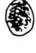

Fig. 8.3   Gumboro disease (IBD). The bursa of Fabricius on the left is normal; that on the right has almost disappeared after infection with Gumboro disease.

Haemorrhages may be seen here and in the muscles of the body, and the kidneys will be swollen, pale and contain urate deposits.

Whilst the disease may not cause a high mortality – usually in the region of 5% – the other effects of the disease can be more serious. The virus, by adversely affecting the bursa of Fabricius, causes profound damage to the whole immunological system of the chicken. The chick may suffer in consequence from other diseases, especially as it may now be unable to get proper protection from vaccines. In many ways it is this last effect which is the most serious one and it will be considered further in the chapter. In the late 1980s a much more virulent form of Gumboro disease became prevalent in many parts of the world and has now spread to virtually all of the large poultry-growing areas. The worst effects have been in broilers and especially cockerels and mortality may reach 40% when the birds are unprotected. Dealing with Gumboro disease involves three procedures. The first is hygiene to the highest standard to minimise or at least delay the likely challenge to succeeding crops. The virus causing Gumboro disease is an extremely persistent one and it is unlikely it will be completely eliminated by cleaning and disinfection. Second, protection is given to the chicks by the use of a live vaccine administered by droplet spray or in the drinking water. A wide range of vaccines of varying strength is available; the choice will be dependent on the degree of the local challenge expected, but at worst it may be necessary to give the vaccine to a broiler flock more than once. Third, there are also inactivated vaccines for use in breeders so that they pass on a strong passive immunity to the chicks that should protect them up to 3–4 weeks of age. Unfortunately, the more virulent forms of the virus break through the maternal immunity much earlier so the chicks may have to be protected from an even earlier age by a 'stronger' vaccine.

There are a number of live and inactivated vaccines available throughout the world but only a limited number may be licensed for use in some countries. This is because it is extremely unwise to use a vaccine which causes such a strong reaction which, whilst it will protect against Gumboro disease, will also cause damage to the immunity system of the bird (termed immunosuppression). The vaccines currently in use in the UK appear capable of controlling infection in young birds, and when given to adults enable a passive immunity to be passed to the chick to last for a time after hatching. Several live inactivated vaccines are now available to give good results.

The infectious stunting syndrome

A new and rather alarming condition was recognised in broilers in the mid-1980s. Known as infectious stunting syndrome (and also malabsorption syndrome and pale bird syndrome) the symptoms are of large-scale stunting in the birds so that, by the time the birds usually reach their normal finishing weight of about 2 kg, up to 20% may weigh only about half this amount. Birds do not die from the disease but they are, needless to say, grossly uneconomic. The affected birds show very poor feathering and the characteristic post-mortem signs are confined to abnormalities of the pancreas.

The disease appears to be due to a virus – it is a transmissible condition showing rapid contagion – and is believed, in the USA, to be an adenovirus for which a vaccine is available. Attempts to identify it as an adenovirus in the UK have so far failed and the only measures one can advise at present are to treat the day-old chicks suspected of carrying the virus with soluble vitamins, electrolytes and broad-spectrum antibiotics. Some of the stunting condition may be due to one or more reoviruses and suitable reovaccines have helped to counteract their condition. It appears that infected breeder flocks produce chicks carrying this virus for a limited period only, similar to viral arthritis.

Clostridial diseases

There is a significant number of clostridial bacteria capable of causing disease on the poultry farm. Clostridial bacteria are a large group which are capable of 'building up' as a problem if the site is kept unhygienically, is overstocked or badly constructed. Some of the diseases of poultry caused by clostridia are malignant oedema (or gangrenous dermatitis), necrotic enteritis and botulism. Clostridial organisms may also be found in association with many other diseases as 'secondaries', for example in yolk sac infection. There is also strong evidence that the weakening of the birds' immunity by Gumboro disease may be the forerunner to certain of these, especially malignant oedema. Clostridia are also serious hatchery pathogens and can cause enormous problems.

Malignant oedema (gangrenous dermatitis)

Malignant oedema is an unpleasant and serious disease of broilers caused by *Clostridium septicum* and *Clostridium perfringens* Type A, which has become more common recently. It occurs towards the end of the growing cycle and may cause massive loss: even up to 50% of the birds. The effect is to cause gangrene of the muscle and of the skin so that the birds in a sense 'fall apart' whilst still alive.

It is often stated and believed that malignant oedema is associated with bad hygiene practices, the re-use of old litter for example and also overstocking and bad environmental conditions. There is probably a measure of truth in this but the disease can certainly occur without any of these being obvious and I have seen its devastating effects in flocks which are kept impeccably. What is known, however, is that it often happens after birds have had their immunity suppressed with diseases, such as Gumboro disease or chicken anaemia virus or there have been other debilitating diseases, such as inclusion body hepatitis (see later in this chapter). Also it should be noted that whilst *Cl. septicum* and *Cl. perfringens* may be the main infective agents with malignant oedema they are by no means the only ones involved: *Staphylococcus aureus* is often the predominating bacteria. Thus, whilst penicillin-G may be the antibiotic of choice to deal with this infection where clostridial organisms are involved, it may be less effective against staphylococcus. It is also important where outbreaks occur to consider carefully the programme for controlling Gumboro disease because outbreaks of this condition so often precede the attacks of malignant oedema. In view of the likelihood that the disease is caused by not only clostridial and staphylococcal organisms, prophylaxis and therapy is best dealt with by using medicines with a broad spectrum of activity and it is usually better to use tetracyclines or amoxycillins rather than penicillin.

Necrotic enteritis

This is also a disease which is more usually found in broilers than in other types of chicken, although not exclusively so. The clostridium involved is *Cl. perfringens* Type C and the condition may lead to a mortality of up to 10%. Lesions are confined to the small intestine, which is grossly inflamed and distended.

This clostridal disease, like others, has often been found in poultry houses with earth or chalk floors where the disease organisms can build up in certain areas which are probably inadequately cleaned or disinfected. Fortunately earth floors are becoming more of a rarity but where they are used it is worth emphasising that they can still be disinfected reasonably with the modern materials available (see Chapter 1). Preventive or curative treatment is effective using appropriate penicillin, tetracyclines or amoxycillin.

Botulism

This is another disease of poultry caused by a clostridium (*Cl. botulinum*) which occurs predominantly in broilers and can cause heavy mortality. Cases of 20% losses in birds near the killing age of 45 days have been seen. The course of this disease is rather different from other clostridia insofar as the organisms multiply in the gut, releasing a toxin which causes paralysis of the muscles, especially of the head and neck.

Fortunately botulism is relatively uncommon. The type of clostridium causing botulism in chickens is *not* the same as that which causes the disease in man. There is no treatment for poultry suffering from this condition but outbreaks are usually associated with dirty, badly managed sites, so that improvements in hygiene are usually essential to further prevention.

Inclusion body hepatitis (IBH)

IBH is a relative newcomer to the poultry field, also mainly associated with broiler chickens. It occurs generally in the period 30–50 days of age. It has no special symptoms except that in a flock which is probably growing very well and is apparently in the best of health, a sudden heavy mortality arises which may give a loss of up to about 10%. Post-mortem signs are usually confined to the liver and kidneys, the former being much enlarged and containing many haemorrhages, whilst the kidneys are also enlarged with haemorrhages throughout. A laboratory examination should be made to confirm the presence of this disease which is caused by a virus.

Fatty liver kidney syndrome (FLKS)

This is an interesting and relatively common disease of chickens between about 7 and 35 days of age. The symptoms are definite; usually there is a rather higher mortality than there should be, and a few birds will be seen lying face downwards and apparently paralysed. The post-morten examination of affected birds shows a pale, swollen liver with haemorrhages, with the heart also pale and the kidneys swollen and usually inflamed. It should be noted that it is predominantly the best birds which are affected by this condition and it is associated with excessive levels of fat deposition.

Cause

It has now been established that FLKS is a disease induced by feeding high levels of wheat or other carbohydrate feed with lower than normal levels of protein so that the ratio between carbohydrate and protein is too wide. It has also been confirmed that if diets containing these incorrect levels are fed, then supplementation of the diet with biotin at levels between 0.05 mg/kg and 0.10 mg/kg of feed will prevent FLKS. Now that this fact is known, the condition is less common but it does occur from time to time due to omission by the compounders of added biotin. It has been stated that biotin is perhaps the most important nutritional factor for poultry. As well as affecting the liver, it has an important influence on the skin, feathers, legs and feet and bones and cartilage. A correct level is vital for the birds' health and development.

Respiratory diseases of chicks

With the increase in the intensity and size of poultry units an enormous surge has occurred in the incidence of respiratory diseases. As a group these are the most important causes of ill-health in poultry in almost all parts of the world. It is unusual nowadays to find respiratory disease in an uncomplicated form. The usual pattern is for one or more primary virus infections, acute or chronic, to be followed by secondary bacterial invaders in which strains of *E. coli* and *Pasturella* usually predominate. Preventive techniques are all-important since the losses from mortality or poor growth and food conversion can be so severe that it may be extremely difficult to stop a catastrophic economic loss.

The approach to preventing losses cannot be generalised because the types of infection and their incidence vary a great deal geographically. If there is a high incidence, say of Newcastle disease and/or infectious bronchitis which are two of the main diseases, a key weapon in the preventive policy would be to protect the birds by vaccination. The strains of vaccine to be used and their frequency of use will depend on the local challenges that predominate and the parental immunity of the chicks. This parental immunity may have been derived from infection in the parent flock or from a suitable vacci-nation policy. As well as protection by vaccination, which will always be concerned with protecting birds from the primary viral agents, there may also be useful ways of protecting the birds against secondary bacterial infections by medicating the stock with antibiotics or chemotherapeutic agents, either in the food or drinking water. Finally, all these measures should be supported by good husbandry, such as the application of warmth, improving the air flow, adding litter and changing lighting systems. We are faced once again with the salient fact that the seriousness of respiratory infections will depend predominantly on the influence of management and housing (Fig 8.4).

Infectious bronchitis

Universally this is the most widely experienced respiratory disease and is caused by a highly contagious virus. There are a substantial number of strains and whilst most primarily affect the respiratory system, there are some varieties, now apparently on the increase in many parts of the world, which also have a serious effect on the kidneys, causing what is known as the uraemic form of the disease.

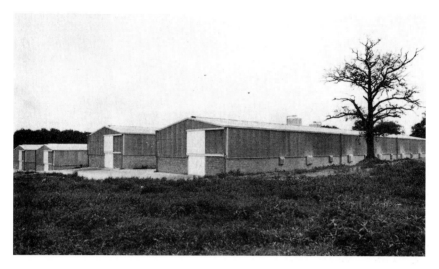

Fig. 8.4   A large deep pit poultry unit with ventilation extracting air from the droppings pit to prevent gases passing into the poultry housing above the pit.

Symptoms

The most noticeable sign in the young chick is a large amount of respiratory noise. Birds sneeze, gasp and shake their head; and in a large flock the best way of detecting early signs is to 'look and listen'. Enter the house very quietly, or if the birds are disturbed by your entry, wait until they are still. If you look you will see their heads shaking and probably an uneven spread of birds. The 'snicking' of the birds will be clearly heard and is almost symptomatic. Early diagnosis is vital because it enables medication to be started immediately. If the disease is allowed to advance unchecked the respiratory noise will usually get worse, with eye-watering, nasal discharge and increasing mortality, followed by secondary infections that take over so that the original infection may be completely masked.

If the only infection is the infectious bronchitis virus, the disease could be over within a week to a fortnight, but it is rare for there to be such a happy outcome. Nevertheless, if the disease is uncomplicated the effect can be mild and recovery can be complete, rather like the common cold in man. What usually happens in practice is that as soon as the birds show signs of sickness they start huddling together and this provides the ideal medium for the propagation of other infections, viral or bacterial, but often apparently dominated by *E. coli*.

In older birds infectious bronchitis can have two profound effects on the female. Infection in the immature female can prevent development of the oviduct, partially or completely, so that the bird will lay few if any eggs. In the other case, if the flock is adult and laying, it will lead to a massive drop in egg production, which may partially recover, but in addition there will tend to be, after a time, the production of poor-quality eggs and eggshells. Eggs are often of strange shapes, the eggshells are ridged and lack pigment and the white of the egg is watery.

When layers are affected egg production will usually fall dramatically and may return to normal over a period of weeks. However, this seldom happens and usually only partial recovery takes place. The economic loss is thus very serious. It is even worse for the poultry breeder because a bronchitis infection during production can not only lower egg numbers and quality but also affect fertility and hatchability adversely. All this together emphasises the importance of giving susceptible birds protection by a complete vaccination programme if there is a fair risk of a challenge with the field virus.

Post-mortem signs in chicks affected with the respiratory form will include the detection of catarrh in the trachea, congested lungs and cloudy air sacs. When the kidneys are affected, they appear considerably enlarged and are white with the deposition of urates. Sometimes urate deposits are seen throughout the body cavities. The effect on the oviduct is to reduce it in size, sometimes so much that it is almost absent, whilst with the mature bird the misshapen ova are diagnostic.

Diagnosis

The symptoms of infectious bronchitis after an incubation period of 1–4 days appear to be so reasonably straightforward that they would allow a clinical diagnosis to be effected without laboratory tests but because the occurrence of the disease is rarely without other intruders, it is often necessary to have samples tested at the laboratory to be certain. For example, the milder forms of Newcastle disease or mycoplasmosis can produce rather similar symptoms. In any case, once the secondary bacteria have invaded to cause damage, specific diagnostic signs will be masked. Thus plenty of use is made of the various tests which are either by virus isolation or by specific antibodies in the sera. The great advantage of having a positive diagnosis done is that whilst it is unlikely that the result will be in time to influence the treatment that will be used in the flock in question, it may be possible to plan or modify future control measures in the light of this information. A more recent problem has been the emergence of a number of different new strains of the infectious bronchitis virus. These 'variants', as they are known, can be identified and it is important to do this wherever indicated so that the appropriate vaccination programme can be carried out. Without this knowledge flocks of birds may be completely vulnerable to infection, having been protected from the 'wrong' strains.

Control

Details of the approach to the control of the disease are given at the end of the section on Newcastle disease because it is best to consider the control of these two similar diseases together.

Newcastle disease (ND)

Just like infectious bronchitis, Newcastle disease tends to occur throughout the world wherever there are large poultry populations. Whilst the first outbreak that was reported and described occurred in Newcastle, England, in 1927, this resulted from an importation of the most virulent form of the disease from the Far East. The first outbreaks that occurred in those days were nearly all extremely virulent and killed off virtually all affected and in-contact birds. Since that time, various other forms of the disease have occurred, many being much milder in extent and others somewhere between the two extremes. At the time of writing the most virulent cases appear to occur in the warmer countries, and the milder cases in the more temperate climates. The last serious outbreak in the UK of really virulent ND started in Essex in 1970 but the so-called Essex 70 strain which could cause almost 100% mortality currently seems to have been replaced by field infections which do not appear to be very much worse than vaccine strains.

In the UK several outbreaks occurred in 1997 in chickens and turkeys, including a substantial number in Ulster, where no vaccine had been used. After good control measures, including vaccination with live and inactivated vaccines, the outbreaks were firstly contained and then eliminated after a few months. It is believed that the outbreaks were due to infected migrating birds of various species entering from Northern Europe.

Symptoms

The incubation period of ND is usually 2–7 days but it may be prolonged for up to 3 weeks. Normally the first signs in a flock are an unusual lassitude and indifference to food and water throughout the flock. The complete lack of the normal reactions of lively birds is quite symptomatic. There may be signs of respiratory distress, some birds apparently struggling for breath, with weird high-pitched 'cries' issuing forth in isolated cases: a symptom which does not seem to occur with any other disease. There is likely also to be a green, watery diarrhoea and the appearance of nervous symptoms which does not occur with the other respiratory diseases. The nervous signs show up as a drooping of either one or both wings, incoordination, falling over and paddling of the legs and twitching and twisting of the neck muscles.

If these three main groups of symptoms are found in a flock then the presence of ND is fairly certain. However, a diagnostic check should always be made and in any case it is unlikely that the pattern would be quite so logically presented as may seem implied; only some of the symptoms might be seen. Confusion can occur with several other diseases; also, if some protection has been afforded by parental immunity or partial vaccination, the end picture would be a very different one. For example, in layers the only effect might be a drop in the egg production and egg quality without a subsequent return to normality. It will already be apparent that confusion with infectious bronchitis could be very easy and there are many more diseases which could be confused with it.

Post-mortem signs

Some or all of the following signs may be seen. The respiratory tract is usually inflamed, the air sacs are cloudy and there are small haemorrhages – known as 'petechiae' – on the heart and especially the proventriculus. There is often a great deal of caseous (dried pus-like) material in the trachea and bronchi and haemorrhages can be seen on the mucous membranes of the respiratory system.

Diagnosis

Clinical symptoms as described, together with the most prominent post-morten signs, may be sufficient to be almost sure of diagnosis but it is nearly always necessary to have laboratory tests done. This may be done by virus isolation and/or serological testing, mostly using the Haemagglutination Inhibition Test.

Control measures

If we start with the chick, in most cases where the disease is prevalent it will be necessary to vaccinate all parent flocks very thoroughly. It is then likely that the chicks will be born with a good immunity. There may not seem, therefore, very much point in an immediate vaccination and, whilst this is not entirely untrue, there are good practical reasons in large flocks to give some protection almost as soon after hatching as possible. One reason is that in large houses of many thousands of birds there will almost certainly be some chicks which do not have an immunity. Thus, an early vaccination will protect them. Furthermore, if an early vaccination is given, it has been found that later vaccinations will cause less stress. The problem of stress cannot be exaggerated. The vaccines now used on chicks by water or spray adminis-tration are very effective but they are live and mildy virulent. Properly used they will cause no harmful effects but if incorrectly or carelessly used they are quite capable of causing a severe reaction which may be followed by secondary infections that can be almost as bad as the disease.

Protection of the birds

Newcastle disease: For Newcastle disease there are three widely used vaccines, two being live vaccines (Hitchner B1 and La Sota) and one an inactivated oil-based vaccine. The first two are administered by spray, drinking water, or occasionally eye-drop, whilst the oil-based vaccine is given by injection. B1 is a safe 'gentle' vaccine which, when given by mass techniques, especially a spray, gives instant protection but protects for only a few weeks. La Sota is a little more stressful but is still mild and will protect for up to 12 weeks in the more mature bird. Now there are additional 'Clone' vaccines with an extremely mild effect but better protection. The oil-based vaccine by injection is most frequently used in the older bird – commonly at the point of lay – and will protect for a laying season but does not give immediate protection. Nevertheless, it seems that within this 'armoury' of vaccines we can usually find the protection needed for any set of circumstances, although in countries where the most virulent forms of Newcastle disease are present, it is usual to have some of the more powerful vaccines available, such as Komarov. These have the disadvantage that they cause very considerable stress on the birds, and hence most countries will not license their use.

Infectious bronchitis: There are three commonly used vaccines to protect birds against infectious bronchitis. These are two live vaccines, the relatively mild Massachusetts type H120, which is used early in life and gives immediate and limited protection, and the H52 which gives a much longer protection and can be used to cover the laying period. Additionally an oil-based inactivated vaccine has been produced which, if given to a bird 3–4 weeks before the laying period, will protect it through the whole of lay. It must be emphasised that full protection must be provided at all stages of development, not only to ensure that the birds throw off any challenge that might cause respiratory disease, but also because of the danger that if a potential layer or breeder contracts the disease during its development, the reproductive organs can be so damaged that egg production will be profoundly affected. Where the disease challenge 'in the field' is complicated by variant strains then it is advisable for these to be identified and if the appropriate vaccines are available to use these. A great deal of development in this area is currently taking place and it is vital to discover which strains are present and to establish whether the vaccines are available to protect the birds.

Table 8.1 sets out certain programmes of protection which can be used either as general routine protection where indicated, or for special emergencies or where there are severe challenges. It is well to stress that even in the presence of Newcastle disease it is possible to spray birds with a large droplet (about 50 microns in diameter or above), and this may arrest the disease on the site since the vaccine particles have a 'blocking' effect by

Table 8.1 Newcastle disease and infectious bronchitis programme by the use of a large particle spray or via drinking water or by injection.

Age	Method	Vaccine Broilers	Breeders/Layers	Remarks
1–4 days General sensitising dose	Spray	B1 and H-120 or similar	B1 and H-120	Helps to reduce stress from subsequent vaccination
Primary vaccination 12–14 days	Spray	B1 and H-120 or similar	B1	No necessity to use both if risk is small
Secondary vaccination 22–28 days	Spray	B1 or La Sota or similar	B1 or La Sota	No necessity to use both if risk is small
35–42 days	Spray	B1 or La Sota or similar	B1 or La Sota	Final vaccination for broilers; unnecessary if low risk
10 weeks	Spray La Sota H-52 in water		La Sota or inactivated and H-52	
Just before point of lay	Spray or injection		La Sota or inactivated for IB and ND	Inactivated oil-based vaccines recommended for this application. La Sota live vaccine will give a much shorter immunity and necessitates revaccination during lay

☐ Spray vaccination is generally more effective than drinking water application provided it is correctly applied. In those flocks in which coli-septicaemia is a major problem spray vaccination can increase this problem and on such premises drinking water application may be used as an alternative

☐ Spray vaccination works in two ways: it induces a rapid rise in antibody and also gives a useful measure of protection on respiratory surfaces themselves, known as 'Local Block'

☐ For boosting during lay, La Sota needs revaccinating after 5 months, but no revaccination is required with inactivated vaccines

☐ La Sota vaccine is not currently licensed for use in the UK

☐ New vaccines are becoming available to protect birds from infectious bronchitis variant viruses giving localised protection via the cells of the respiratory mucous membranes. In this connection the virtues of the large particle size spray, such as the 'Turbair' (see Fig. 8.5), should be emphasised, as compared with the small particle aerosol which is best *not* used. The latter penetrates deeply into the respiratory system and can cause a serious reaction. A method of using infectious bronchitis vaccine at day-old – if desired in the hatchery – has been developed by using the large particle spray with considerable success as it gives a minimum of reaction and a maximum of protection.

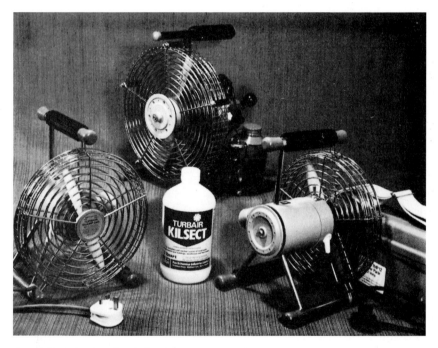

Fig. 8.5   The 'Turbair' droplet sprayer can be used for vaccination, insecticides and disinfectant.

Mycoplasma infection (CRD)

Mycoplasma are a group of organisms that cause a great deal of disease in the animal population. They are not dissimilar to, but are still quite distinct from bacteria, being smaller. They are also free living which distinguishes them from viruses.

In livestock these organisms are mostly associated with respiratory diseases and the long-known poultry disease of 'chronic respiratory disease' is primarily caused by *Mycoplasma gallisepticum*. The usual signs of the disease in a flock are sneezing, snicking and coughing, inflamed and running eyes and swelling of the sinuses of the face. The lesions to be seen in the bird are likely to be confined to the respiratory tract and will consist of varying degrees of inflammation and exudates in the tract, lungs and the air sacs. The disease in itself can cause some mortality and loss of productivity but it is very often a precursor to the other respiratory diseases. It is more serious in its effects on the younger bird than the older one.

Control

Mycoplasmosis is a less contagious and less acutely virulent disease than the worst forms of Newcastle disease or infectious bronchitis. There is no vaccine to prevent it but nevertheless it may be controlled very effectively in several ways. The most satisfactory way is to build up an entire breeding enterprise that is free of disease by blood testing and elimination of infected birds. There are good serological tests and this procedure has been so successful that most breeding stock in the UK and USA and western Europe are now free of *M. gallisepticum* infection. There are also several antibiotics that will successfully control the disease so these may be used in conjunction with a blood testing programme. Because the organisms can be transmitted from hen to chick via the egg, it is also recommended, in infected breeder flocks, to treat the hatching eggs by dipping them in suitable solutions containing anti–mycoplasmal drugs.

A related mycoplasma, *M. synoviae*, is also a widespread cause of disease. Whilst it is primarily a cause of lameness, due to the inflammation it causes in leg joints, it also retards growth and causes respiratory infections. Control measures are similar to those for *M. gallisepticum*.

Infectious laryngotracheitis (ILT)

Infection laryngotracheitis is a highly virulent virus disease whose incidence is world-wide but is confined to certain areas. Symptoms are usually an extremely serious respiratory involvement with great distress exhibited by the birds as they struggle for breath, accompanied by coughing and rattling, and often with the bird depositing bloody mucus. There may also be less acute forms of the disease which are less severe but otherwise similar. Post-mortem examination of birds with ILT shows severe inflammation of the larynx and trachea with bloody, cheesy 'clots' virtually filling the trachea. The virus that causes ILT does not affect any other organs and the birds die of asphyxiation.

Diagnosis can be made with a considerable degree of certainty from the symptoms, post-mortem picture and history but it is advisable to have a laboratory check on specimens and if necessary seek virus isolation or serological tests.

Treatment and prevention

There is no medicine available that will affect the virus of ILT and the only effect of treatment with antibiotics and vitamin supplements will be to assist the birds' resistance to secondary infection. There are, however, good vaccines available to prevent the disease, the modern ones being the modified live virus which may be given by the eye-drop route.

It is important to emphasise that 'recovered' birds may remain as carriers of the infection for the rest of their lives. Thus is an eradication programme it is best to start by depopulating the entire site and then follow through with a rigorous cleaning and disinfection programme. This is also one case at least where it would be advisable to leave the premises empty for a few weeks after the disinfection programme has been completed.

Avian rhino tracheitis (ART)

This is also known as turkey rhino tracheitis and swollen head syndrome. It is a pneumovirus disease of turkeys and chicken, affecting all stock from about 2 weeks of age. The disease is characterised by swellings in the corner of the eyes, tracheitis and markedly swollen sinuses in the head. The disease will cause a severe effect on the performance of layers and breeders and in young growers or broilers will lead to secondary infections with *E. coli* and *Pasteurella*.

Treatment can be instituted with broad-spectrum antibiotics; prevention is achieved by a programme of live and inactivated vaccines.

Infectious coryza (roup)

A bacterium *Haemophilus gallinarum* can cause a disease in poultry which is similar to the common cold in man. The symptoms are acute, leading to general inflammation, swelling and discharges around and from the eyes and nose. It does not appear to be a very serious problem nowadays in intensive units but vaccines are made which are effective in preventing it. It may be treated with antibiotics.

Internal parasites of chickens

Coccidiosis

Coccidiosis is undoubtedly the most important parasitic disease of the domestic chicken and yet, because of the successful development of medicines and vaccines to prevent and treat the condition, it is no longer a disease to be feared. Nevertheless, because it is always a potential threat which can cause serious loss it is essential that the poultryman knows when to suspect it and what to do in an emergency. He should also be aware of the range of medicines and vaccines available and how they may be effectively used.

Coccidiosis of chickens is caused by protozoa (single-celled parasites) which live in the lining (epithelium) of the intestine. Those affecting chickens are of the species *Eimeria*. The life-cycle of the various species in the chicken is as follows. There is a massive multiplication of the coccidia (known as schizogony) and sexual multiplication (known as gametogony) within the chicken; then a stage of development takes place outside the host in which the eggs that are shed in sexual development reach a stage when they can infect other chickens, though they do not multiply. These are known as oocysts.

There are six main strains of *Eimeria* species which can cause diseases of the intestines in chickens. Each species causes rather different symptoms because each has a different favoured site within the intestine. For example, the most common *Eimeria* are *E. tenella*, which affects only the caecal tubes and *E. necatrix*, which mainly affects the middle and lower intestines.

Symptoms

The overall symptoms may be one or more of the following: bloody droppings, high mortality, general droopiness, emaciation, a marked drop in feed consumption, diarrhoea and reduced egg production in layers. A proper diagnosis should be made by a veterinary laboratory.

Treatment and control of coccidiosis

Outbreaks of coccidiosis which occur may be treated with sulphonamides or combinations of sulphonamides and pyrimidines or amprolium, all given in the drinking water. Sulphamezathine or sulphaquinoxaline are usually given at 0.1% and 0.4% respectively in the drinking water for 5–7 days.

A wide range of coccidiostats is used to prevent the disease during the growing period. At the present time in broiler feeds some of the most popular coccidiostats are based on monensin and arprinocid and also halofuginone, clopidol, robenidine, diclazuril and amprolium + ethopabate; this list is by no means exhaustive. Changes in medicines are appropriate by careful planning to prevent resistance developing. Certain coccidiostats must also be withdrawn a specified number of days before birds are slaughtered to ensure there are no residues in the carcass.

Because of this it may be necessary to use two anti-coccidial agents, even in the short life of a broiler, as it is risky to try and dispense with any prevention during the last 5–7 days of growth. Replacement birds should not be given an agent that completely destroys the parasites since no immunity develops. In a more recent approach to dealing with coccidiosis in birds being reared for laying or breeding, vaccines have been produced and one administration is sufficient within a few days of hatching. Coccidiostats are still preferred for broilers as they tend to be more cost-effective.

Coccidial immunity

It is especially important with the disease of coccidiosis to know how immunity develops. If birds are to achieve immunity they must ingest a sufficient number of oocysts to produce some infection. These oocysts then go through several life cycles and multiply. Following exposure to a sufficient number of oocysts the bird will then become resistant to the disease. Immunity must be established for each individual species of coccidia because there is no cross-immunity and thus birds can become immune to one species of coccidia yet still be vulnerable to others. Also, immunity is not permanent; it can be lost if the environment of the bird does not provide a sufficient level of re-exposure. In certain tests, loss of immunity was demonstrated within as short a period as 10 weeks.

Two principles are used to achieve the gradual production of immunity as a means of controlling coccidiosis. The first is by the use of medicines or vaccine at low levels to reduce the severity of natural exposure and the second is deliberate seeding of the litter with coccidia to provide a controlled exposure; it is much safer and more reliable to use the former measures. With both of these methods it is possible to have an inadequate exposure, lending to a resultant deficiency in immunity, or an excessive exposure leading to losses from the disease.

Blackhead (histomoniasis)

Blackhead is another disease caused by a protozoan parasite, this one being called *Histomonas meleagridis*. Whilst it is primarily a disease of turkeys it may also affect young chickens in which the disease is mild. The symptoms include watery, yellowish diarrhoea, lethargy, weakness, and loss of appetite. Post-mortem examination shows a marked inflammation, usually with cheesy cores, in the lumen of the caeca; on the liver a number of circular, yellowish-green depressions or ulcers about 12 mm in diameter may be observed.

There are a number of excellent drugs to prevent or cure blackhead; for example dimetridiazole, nifursol and nitrothiazoles and unizole. The occurrence of blackhead in chickens indicates a need to improve hygiene and eliminate intestinal worm parasites since their eggs may carry the blackhead parasites.

The tapeworm (*Davainea proglottina*)

Affected birds lose weight and are listless, breathing is rapid and feathers are ruffled and dry. In laying birds there is reduced egg production. At post mortem the intestinal mucosa may be thickened and haemorrhagic and the tapeworms are seen. For development of the life-cycle the intermediate hosts such as snails and earthworms, have to be present. Specific treatment should be used where the worms are found. Understandably, infection only takes place under extensive or semi-intensive conditions.

The large roundworm (*Ascaridia galli*)

This is a large worm up to 80 mm in length which causes loss of condition, reduced egg production in layers and can even cause death if infection is heavy. Retarded growth, listlessness and diarrhoea are the clearest symptoms. At post mortem the large roundworms can be seen in the middle part of the small intestine. The disease is uncommon under hygienic conditions but certainly occurs if the litter is wet and overcrowded.

The hairworm (*Capillaria*)

The hairworm is a small parasite which affects the upper part of the alimentary tract, causing diarrhoea, weakness, reduced egg production and anaemia. Affected birds are listless, weak and lose weight. Hygienic measures and treatment are as for the other worms.

The caecal worm (*Heterakis gallinae*)

This is a worm about 10 mm size which develops in the caeca and affects chickens and turkeys. Perhaps its most important 'function' is as a transmitter of the parasite causing blackhead (histomoniasis).

Treatment
There are a range of specific treatments to control roundworms and tapeworms, e.g. flubendazole and the piperazines.

External parasites

Poultry can be infested with a variety of external parasites, such as lice, fleas and various forms of mites, e.g. red mite, the depluming mite and scaly leg mite. These mites all burrow into various parts of the birds' skin and create considerable damage. The presence of all these conditions is rather uncommon under modern intensive management and if general standards of hygiene are high it is doubtful if they will be seen at all. External parasites are more commonly associated with older birds and old-fashioned systems of continuous production. If they do occur, then it is advisable to deal with them energetically as they will have a highly debilitating effect on the birds and may also be associated with the spread of other diseases.

Treatment will depend on the administration (Fig. 8.6) of one of the effective products which are listed later in Table 8.2. Of course it need hardly be emphasised that if birds are badly infested, especially with mites, they should be culled, as they are unlikely to respond very effectively to treatment and they will remain as a serious source of infection.

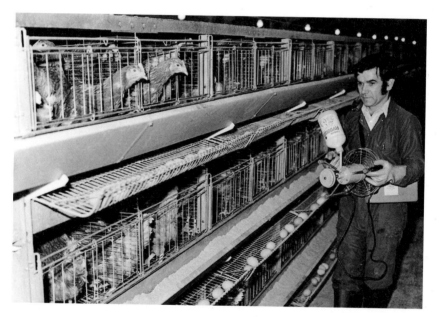

Fig. 8.6   Pyrethrins in oil being aplied in a three-tier cage unit through the Turbair Flydowner 12 battery-powered ULV sprayer for insect control. Birds are not disturbed, due to the low noise level of the sprayer and unobtrusive nature of the fine spray.

Important viral diseases principally of young chickens

Viral arthritis (tenosynovitis)

A widespread form of viral arthritis is quite common in broiler chickens from about 4 weeks onwards. The signs are of serious lameness in the birds, coupled with poor growth rates and bad food conversion efficiences. In the affected birds the flexor tendon sheaths running along the posterior of the tarsometatarsal bones are seen to be swollen, giving the shanks a very enlarged appearance. The sheaths of the gastrocnemius tendons just above the hocks are also swollen. In advanced cases the tendons themselves may frequently rupture. At post mortem the sheaths can be seen to be oedematous, looking almost like gelatin in appearance. There is usually no pus in the inflamed tissues and the remainder of the bird appears almost normal.

A tentative diagnosis on the basis of the clinical signs can usually be made but confirmation depends upon viral isolation and identification.

There seems little doubt that the virus causing this condition is widely spread among the world's poultry industries but only certain broiler flocks are without maternal immunity and are challenged. Thus, the practical incidence of the disease is quite limited. There is no cure for the condition but when flocks are affected the administration of an antibiotic with a wide spectrum of activity plus soluble vitamin preparations is a justified veterinary procedure in order to limit the effect of the disease, guard against secondaries, such as staphylococci and clostridia, and help to overcome the effects of inappetence and poor growth. Increasing use is being made of vaccines in order to artificially immunise breeders.

Epidemic tremor (infectious avian encephalomyelitis (IAE))

Epidemic tremor is caused by a virus of chickens leading to nervous signs and symptoms in young birds. Whilst birds of all ages can be infected it is only in birds up to about 8 weeks of age that the characteristic nervous signs are normally seen. In laying birds an attack causes a drop in egg production of about 10%, which is soon over, but a drop in hatchability also occurs.

Affected chicks show incoordinated movements, falling, collapsing then becoming prostrate and finally dying. If the chick is picked up and rested in the palm of the hand the tremors of the muscle, which are quite characteristic of the disease, may be felt. Usually about 10–15% of the flock are affected and most of them die, although a few make a complete recovery.

A definite diagnosis is made on microscopic examination of the brain and central nervous system where specific changes take place.

Route of infection

The virus infects chicks in two ways: the first route is from the dam to the chick via the ovaries; the second is entry after hatching via the mouth or respiratory system. If chicks are infected via the ovary, they contract the disease within about 7 days of hatching. If the chicks are infected by the oral route, they will become diseased from about 3 weeks onwards.

Control

Fortunately excellent live vaccines are now available to control epidemic tremor. The usual procedure undertaken is to vaccinate breeders to protect them against falls in egg production and hatchability and also to prevent the transfer of infection to their chicks. Vaccination is given between 10 and 16 weeks of age, provided it is done within this period, protection should be satisfactory for the rest of the bird's life.

Chicken anaemia virus (CAV)

Chicken anaemia virus is also known as 'blue wing', infectious anaemia, haemorrhagic syndrome, or anaemia dermatitis syndrome. Chicks contract this disease from an infected parent flock. The effect on the chicks is extremely serious, causing haemorrhage, especially in the wing: hence the synonym 'blue wing'. It is seen most commonly in broilers from 7–10 days of age and leads to very serious immunosuppression and necrotic dermatitis results. Fortunately, the disease is readily prevented by vaccination.

Marek's disease and lymphoid leucosis

Both Marek's disease (Fig. 8.7) and lymphoid leucosis are very important conditions leading to neoplasia (tumours) in chickens and caused by two groups of viruses. Marek's disease is caused by a strongly cell-associated herpesvirus, whilst leucosis is caused by some of the so-called RNA tumour virus group of oncornaviruses. The major manifestations of both diseases are lymphoid neoplasia but in other respects the two conditions differ widely.

Marek's disease was one of the most serious causes of loss in poultry before the relatively recent introduction of vaccines which has enabled its very successful control. It is a disease which causes proliferation of the lymphoid tissue, affecting most organs and tissues but especially the peripheral nerves. It affects chickens most commonly between 12 and 24 weeks of age, although it does occur occasionally in chickens from 6 weeks of age and sometimes, but rarely, in birds older than 24 weeks. The incubation period may vary from as little as 3 weeks to several months. There is one form of

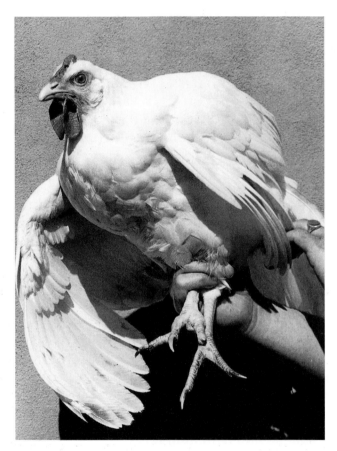

Fig. 8.7   Typical case of Marek's disease, showing paralysis of one wing.

Marek's disease which is known as *acute Marek's*; this causes a very high mortality: up to 30% is quite common, and on occasions even as much as 80%. The disease may proceed in two ways: there may be a quick peak of mortality, rapidly falling away to almost nothing over a period of a few weeks or, alternatively, it may reach a peak quite quickly and then continue without much change for months. Only a proportion of birds may show nervous signs of paralysis.

The alternative and, until recently, the more common form is that known as *classical Marek's* disease. Mortality is usually less, rarely exceeding 10–15%. In some cases mortality proceeds only for a few weeks and in others it may go on for many months. The symptoms differ widely depending on which nerves are affected. Most often there is a progressive paralysis of the wings and legs. Badly affected birds cannot stand and, characteristically, birds are found lying on their sides with one leg stretched forward and the other held behind. In other cases the neck may be twisted, or the respiratory system may be involved, or even the intestines.

Post–mortem signs are of diffuse lymphomatous enlargements of one or more organs or tissues: most often the liver, gonads, spleen, kidneys, lungs, proventriculus and heart. Sometimes the lymphomas also arise in the skin associated with feather follicles and also in the skeletal muscles. In younger birds the liver enlargement is usually moderate in extent but in adults the greatly enlarged liver may appear identical to that in lymphoid leucosis.

Control

There is no treatment for Marek's disease. Control depends on the rearing of young stock in isolation from older birds, the use of genetically resistant stock wherever possible, and above all else, by vaccination. There are several types of vaccine: either modified field strains of Marek's disease virus, or a turkey herpes virus which is a virus antigenically closely related to Marek's disease virus and which is present in most turkey flocks; it is not pathogenic to turkeys or chickens and can be used for vaccination.

There are two forms of the vaccines produced. In one form the vaccine is used in association with the cells and in the other the vaccines are freeze-dried. There is no evidence as to which is definitely the best and both can be recommended. The freeze-dried vaccine, which can be kept in an ordinary refrigerator, is much easier to store and handle than the cell-associated form which must be kept in liquid nitrogen containers at $-100°C$. However, some poultrymen consider the immunity derived from the cell-associated form to be better, perhaps because rather greater care must be taken in its handling.

All vaccines are normally used only once, at 1 day old, and this is most conveniently given at the hatchery. Within a week a reasonable level of protection is obtained and this lasts a lifetime. In the last year or two there have been some unfortunate 'breakdowns' in properly vaccinated flocks. There is no evidence that this is due to any fault in the existing advice or techniques but it is a warning that correct methods of administration must be used. Such has been the concern in the poultry industry about the 'breakdowns' that some organisations are now advising a second vaccination at about 2 weeks of age. The actual choice of vaccine programme must depend on the expected local challenge that is likely.

Leucosis

There are several different forms of avian leucosis. The commonest is lymphoid leucosis, in which there is usually an enlargement of the liver which is so grossly overgrown that it extends the full length of the abdominal cavity, whilst tumours may also affect many other organs of the body, the most common sites being the spleen, kidney and bursa of Fabricius. Another type is erythroid leucosis, which causes a serious anaemia due to the proliferation of excessive numbers of immature red blood cells. The liver, spleen and bone marrow become cherry red in this form. In contrast, in myeloid leucosis there is tumour formation in the liver and spleen, the liver often assuming the appearance of Morocco leather with a granular texture, due to the presence of a large number of discrete and nodular tumours of a chalky or cheesy consistency.

These lesions are all caused by a group of closely related RNA tumour viruses. Virus strains produce predominantly one form of leucosis but many will, in addition, produce lymphoid leucosis. The viruses can be identified by the presence of a group of specific antigens using the Cefal test.

The course of the disease

Most commercial poultry have some measure of infection with certain groups of the leucosis viruses. Recent breakdowns in flocks from Marek's disease have indicated the need for the additional use of the so-called Rispen's strain of vaccine virus in day-old chicks, in combination with the other procedures. Advice may be sought from the manufacturers as to the best programme to prevent this serious disease. The viruses are excreted in the droppings and the saliva and can readily infect in-contact birds. Also, a proportion of eggs are also infected, transferring the virus through to the chick. Chicks receiving their infection through the eggs become tolerant to the virus and do not produce antibodies, whereas those infected after hatching respond with the production of viral antibodies. Chicks tolerant to the virus are more likely to succumb to disease and if they do not they shed viruses in the eggs more consistently than chickens with circulating anti-body. Lymphoid leucosis is the main form of disease developing after infection with leucosis virus. It is evident, however, that only about 2% of chickens die from lymphoid leucosis.

Control

There is no treatment and, because the infection is transmitted through the egg, management and hygiene methods are unable to control the disease. However, the viruses are not highly contagious and it is relatively easy to prevent infection of a flock from outside. If it is possible to free flocks from infection it is possible to maintain them and their progeny free of infection.

Genetic selection of stock resistant to infection with leucosis viruses creates a population resistant to infection with leucosis viruses and also reduces the number of birds capable of supporting infection.

Fowl pox

Fowl pox is a virus infection of the pox group which causes lesions in the head and mouth of the bird. It is also possible to find lesions on the legs and on mucous membranes such as the cloaca. The lesions on the head and comb are usually wart-like in nature, whilst those which occur in the mouth are 'diphtheritic' and have the appearance of a cheesy membrane. The general symptoms depend on the area of the body affected. The birds appear dull and when the mouth is affected they may have difficulty in breathing and eating.

When the virus attacks the mucous membranes of the nasal and buccal cavities mortality can be as high as 40–50%. The virus causes a marked increase in the output of mucus and this is sometimes referred to as 'wet pox'. The less serious skin form of the disease does not lead to high mortality but can cause a reduced egg production in laying birds.

Diagnosis and treatment

The symptoms are usually clear enough to make a diagnosis of the disease, although if there are doubts a veterinary laboratory can confirm.

It is not easy to treat affected birds but it is possible to remove the diphtheritic membranes from the mouth and the surrounding area and then treat with antiseptics and emollients. Prevention can be achieved by using a live pox vaccine which can be administered by wing web or feather follicle application. Fowl pox is a relatively uncommon condition in temperate areas under intensive conditions but remains as a common complaint in warm climates where the systems usually lack good hygiene.

Egg drop syndrome 1976 (EDS '76)

For several years it has been known that a variety of viruses, the so-called adenoviruses, can infect chickens. Whilst they may have an effect at any time of life the most serious strains cause sudden and prolonged falls in egg production and a profound effect on egg and shell quality. One particular strain first caused problems in 1976 in broiler breeder parents and has since been designated EDS '76. The condition has also spread to other adult birds but it is in breeders that the effect has been most serious. The syndrome has shown itself in a number of forms. There may be a failure to peak production or there may be gradual or sudden drops in egg production. The egg production of an affected flock may or may not return to normal. There is also a tendency for lowered hatchability, poor eggshell quality and loss of colour. Diagnosis of this condition requires expert examination since the symptoms can readily be confused with those of infectious bronchitis and Newcastle disease and perhaps other adenoviruses and infectious avian encephalomyelitis. A vaccine has now been produced which has been found to be capable of giving satisfactory protection, e.g. Nobi-Vac EDS '76 vaccine (Intervet Laboratories).

Pullet disease ('blue comb', 'monocytosis')

Pullet disease was once a very common condition of birds affecting them soon after they had come into production. It has all the signs of a viral infection but no virus has been identified. The symptoms are usually a marked fall in egg production together with inappetence and lethargy. Some birds may be found dead, dying too quickly to show symptoms, but in most, and especially later cases in the course of the disease, death is preceded by a short period of illness during which purple-coloured combs and wattles are the most noticeable feature, together with diarrhoea and an extremely dejected appearance.

Post-mortem signs are especially associated with abnormalities in the kidneys which are usually grossly enlarged with crystalline urate deposits. There are also degenerative changes of the birds' ovaries and a general congestion of the carcass, including a patchy discoloration of the pectoral muscles.

The only useful treatment is to administer tetracyclines in the drinking water, ensuring that this is freely available to all the birds. Restriction of food intake may be beneficial for a time and a 'traditional' remedy is to mix in with the diet 10–20% of molasses and feed the whole diet wet.

Two classical bacterial diseases of chickens

Avian tuberculosis

Avian tuberculosis is a disease caused by the bacterium *Mycobacterium tuberculosis avium*. It is a contagious disease passed on by contact via the droppings of infected birds.

The disease normally affects older birds when there is a progressive loss of weight ('going light' as it used to be termed). The birds become unthrifty and the muscles of the breast are reduced in size, exposing the sternum or breast bone. Appetite usually remains normal until the terminal stage of the disease. There may be some lameness and swelling of the joints and the comb and wattles appear pale in colour.

Post-mortem examination reveals lesions which appear as yellowish-white caseous nodules in the liver, spleen and intestines. Laboratory examination can confirm the presence of the disease.

No treatment is effective and the disease is best dealt with by good culling of the affected birds combined with a complete depopulation of the house and subsequent disinfection.

Fowl cholera (avian pasteurellosis)

Fowl cholera is caused by a bacterium, *Pasteurella multicida*, and can be a very serious cause of disease in many parts of the world. Infection occurs by the respiratory or alimentary route which contaminates water, soil and feed. There is an incubation period of 4–10 days and the severity of the condition depends very much on the 'stress' imposed on the birds by poor ventilation, overcrowding and so on. Symptoms in the most acute cases include sudden death in large numbers with signs of cyanosis (purple or mauve colouring) and swelling of the comb and wattles. In the less acute stages there is swelling of the joints and legs causing lameness. Affected birds do not eat or drink and have difficulty in breathing. A thick nasal discharge will be seen together with a greenish-yellow diarrhoea. Mortality may be very high, even up to 90%. Diagnosis is made on the basis of the symptoms and on isolation of the organism.

Treatment may be instituted by using antibiotics and medicines and prevention can be effected by vaccination. The incidence of tuberculosis and fowl cholera has decreased markedly under hygienic intensive conditions and with the better understanding of these diseases and the use of good medicines and vaccines both diseases may be expected to diminish in seriousness worldwide.

Mycotoxicosis

Chicks of all ages may be affected with forms of the fungus-induced disease known as mycotoxicosis. This is really a group of diseases which arise from toxins released by moulds found in certain feedstuffs or in the litter of the poultry house. Symptoms are usually indefinite but there may be a number of birds off-colour, obviously sick, droopy, eating and drinking little or nothing and several will die. Post-mortem signs are mostly confined to the liver which may be congested in acute cases or, in chronic cases, pale or yellowish-brown in colour and hard. Confirmation of the involvement of a mycotoxin requires detailed microscopic examination of the liver and the feed the birds have been receiving.

There is no specific treatment but the administration of vitamins, especially B vitamins in the water, is warranted in an attempt to reduce some of the effects of the toxins. A number of chemicals are currently available for the treatment of either the food or the litter and housing, e.g. kemin.

Table 8.2 The health of poultry: a summary of diseases, prevention and treatment.

Disease	Prevention	Treatment
Adenovirus	Vaccine may protect against one type EDS '76 (egg drop syndrome 1976)	Non-specific measures such as vitamin, mineral and electrolyte mixtures and often broad-spectrum antibiotics may assist in the bird's recovery, e.g. chlortetracycline or amoxycillin
Aspergillosis	Avoid all damp litter and nest material	Treat whole environment with a disinfectant active against fungi
Avian clostridial diseases	Hygienic measures within and around buildings require to be improved and there is a need for an improved disinfection and fumigation programme	Soluble penicillin or amoxycillin in drinking water
Avian mycoplasmosis (CRD)	Normally eliminated by blood testing and removal of reactors. Also by medication with antibiotics such as Lincospectin, tylosin or rovamycin	Similar to preventives
Avian pasteurellosis	Vaccination by injection of Pasteurella vaccine	Amoxycillin. Chlortetracycline. Oxytetracycline
Avian rhino tracheitis	Live and inactivated vaccines. Protect young birds and breeders	Improve ventilation and treat secondaries with broad-spectrum antibiotics
Chicken anaemia virus	Vaccination by administration in the drinking water or by injection	Soluble vitamins, especially Vitamin K-fortified preparations
Coccidiosis	Medication of ration with a variety of coccidiostats, e.g. Elancoban, salinomycin, clopidol, narasin, Cycostat and diclazuril, nicarbazin	Various sulphonamides and potentiated sulpha drugs and Paracox vaccine

Table 8.2 Continued

Disease	Prevention	Treatment
E. coli infections	*E. coli* is usually a secondary infection; thus prevent primary disease with vaccination, therapy or good husbandry. Useful medicines are potentiated sulphonamides, Lincospectin and neomycin	Chlortetracycline hydrochloride. Lincospectin. Amoxycillin. Enrofloxacin
Fatty liver and kidney syndrome (FLKS)	Ensure that protein and carbohydrate ratio is correct and that the ration is sufficient in biotin and other Vitamin B elements	Administer water soluble vitamin preparation fortified with biotin
Fowl pox	Vaccination effectively prevents	Administer non-specific broad-spectrum antibiotics for secondary infections
Gangrenous dermatitis	Usually associated with broilers after early Gumboro disease challenge so vaccination against latter assists. Do not use 'old' litter or overstock, and ensure perfect disinfection between crops	Soluble penicillin or amoxycillin in water. Amoxycillin together with soluble fortified vitamins
Gumboro disease (infectious bursal diseases)	Gumboro disease vaccines. Choice depends on virulence of virus	Treat for secondary infections with vitamin/antibiotic preparations
Histomoniasis (blackhead)	Dimetridiazole and other nitrothiazoles	As prevention, and nifursol
Inclusion body hepatitis (IBH)	Gumboro vaccination may assist in prevention as Gumboro disease appears to predispose to infection of IBH	Non-specific measures including broad-spectrum antibiotics and vitamins, especially fat-soluble vitamins
Infectious avian encephalomyelitis (epidemic tremor)	A variety of live vaccines administered in drinking water at an age of about 15 weeks	No specific treatment
Infectious bronchitis	Vaccination. Primary with H-120 spray or drinking water, continue for rearers with H-52 in coarse spray or drinking water or use inactivated injectable vaccine	To curb secondary infections, use broad-spectrum anti-biotics
Infectious laryngotracheitis	Vaccination by individual ocular or nasal drop or in spray	Non-specific broad-spectrum antibiotics and vitamins

Table 8.2   Continued

Disease	Prevention	Treatment
Insect infestation	A wide range of materials exist for dealing with flies, lice, beetles and crawling insects which are especially liable to infest poultry houses due to their warmth and their cavity construction. Many are organophosphorus compounds	
Marek's disease	Vaccinate day-old chicks by intramuscular route. With appropriate vaccine, e.g. turkey or chicken herpes or Rispens'	No specific treatment but vitamin and mineral preparations added to drinking water may assist birds. Also treatment for any intercurrent infection, such as coccidiosis or secondary bacterial infections
Necrotic enteritis	Improved hygiene including phenolic disinfectants and penicillin in feed at a level of 40 g per tonne	Soluble penicillin in water or broad-spectrum antibiotic, e.g. oxytetracycline hydrochloride soluble
Newcastle disease (notifiable in UK)	Variety of vaccines protect, e.g. Hitchner B1 and La Sota, by droplet or water medication largely for young or growing stock, and inactivated oil-adjuvant vaccines by injection, primarily for layers or breeders (In some countries, e.g. UK, only some vaccines are legal and a slaughter policy may be followed)	No effective treatment against virus of Newcastle disease but treatment for secondaries as under *E. coli* infections
Perosis	Balanced ration sufficient, especially in manganese, other minerals and available phosphorus	As prevention, administering extra vitamins and minerals in soluble form
Roundworms	Normal hygiene measures during and between batches of chicken on litter	Flubendazole and piperazine preparations
Salmonellosis	Prevention relies on good hygiene, correct feeding practice and testing by veterinary diagnostic laboratories for the organisms. Certain vaccines also available, e.g. Salenvac for enteriditis	Enrofloxacin. Amoxycillin. Neomycin. Sulpha medicines

Table 8.2 Continued

Disease	Prevention	Treatment
Stress	Mixtures of vitamins, minerals and electrolytes, which may, on veterinary advice, incorporate an antibiotic	
Viral arthritis (tenosynovitis)	Vaccines	Broad-spectrum antibiotics
Yolk sac infection	Hygienic measures in hatchery, breeding farms and chick accommodation	Non-specific broad-spectrum antibiotics

Index